GARLAND STUDIES ON

# THE ELDERLY IN AMERICA

*edited by*
**STUART BRUCHEY**
ALLAN NEVINS PROFESSOR EMERITUS
COLUMBIA UNIVERSITY

# NUTRITION SUPPORT TO ELDERLY WOMEN

### INFLUENCE ON DIET QUALITY

MICHELLE B. PIERCE

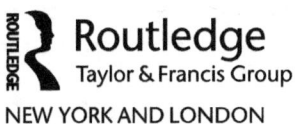

First published in 2000 by Garland Publishing Inc.

Published 2016 by Routledge
711 Third Avenue, New York, NY 10017, USA
2 Park Square, Milton Park, Abingdon, Oxfordshire OX14 4RN

First issued in paperback 2016

*Routledge is an imprint of the Taylor & Francis Group, an informa business*

Copyright © 2000 by Michelle B. Pierce

All rights reserved. No part of this book may be reprinted or reproduced or utilized in any form or by any electronic, mechanical, or other means, now known or hereafter invented, including photocopying and recording, or in any information storage or retrieval system, without permission in writing from the publishers.

**Library of Congress Cataloging-in-Publication Data**
Pierce, Michelle B., 1958–
    Nutrition support to elderly women : influence on diet quality / Michelle B. Pierce.
       p. cm. — (Garland studies on the elderly in America)
    Includes bibliography and index.
    ISBN 0-8153-3812-0 (alk. paper)
    1. Aged women—Nutrition—Social aspects. 2. Aged women—Diseases—Nutritional aspects. I. Title. II. Series.
RC952.5 .P52  2000
613.2'084'6—dc21                                                    99-055080

ISBN 13: 978-1-138-97735-8 (pbk)
ISBN 13: 978-0-8153-3812-3 (hbk)

# Dedication

To the memory of my Grandfather
Edward B. Bitzer, Sr.
You were with me, from beginning to end.

# Contents

| | |
|---|---|
| List of Tables | ix |
| List of Figures | xi |
| Acknowledgments | xiii |
| | |
| Chapter 1: Introduction | 3 |
| Social Relationships | 4 |
| Prior Research | 7 |
| Stress | 18 |
| Conclusion | 21 |
| Objectives | 22 |
| Overview of Book | 23 |
| | |
| Chapter 2: Methods | 25 |
| Pilot Studies | 25 |
| Subject Selection | 27 |
| Phase I: Focus Groups and Key Informant Interviews | 29 |
| Phase II: Structured Interviews | 38 |
| | |
| Chapter 3: Description of the Subjects | 47 |
| Demographics | 47 |
| Health | 51 |
| Nutritional Risk | 58 |
| Social Anchorage | 59 |
| Conclusion | 62 |
| | |
| Chapter 4: Nutrition-Related Concerns and Proffered Help | 65 |

| | |
|---|---|
| The Issues | 65 |
| Helping Behaviors | 74 |
| Conclusion | 82 |
| | |
| Chapter 5: Nutrition-Related Social Support | 85 |
| Modified Diets | 86 |
| Food and Meal Procurement | 100 |
| Comparison with Support Models | 113 |
| | |
| Chapter 6: Food Intake and Dietary Adequacy | 117 |
| Food Patterns | 117 |
| Nutrient Intakes | 121 |
| Implications | 131 |
| Dietary Quality | 132 |
| Discussion and Conclusions | 136 |
| | |
| Chapter 7: Functional Status, Social Support and Dietary Quality | 139 |
| Buffering Model | 140 |
| Relationships between Functional Status, Social Support and Dietary Quality | 145 |
| Satisfaction with Food Acquisition Support | 163 |
| Discussion | 164 |
| | |
| Chapter 8: Conclusions | 167 |
| Summary of Results | 167 |
| Discussion | 172 |
| Limitations | 175 |
| Recommendations | 177 |
| Conclusion | 183 |
| | |
| Appendices | 185 |
| References | 211 |
| Author Index | 229 |
| Subject Index | 235 |

# Tables

| | | |
|---|---|---|
| 1. | Progression of research | 26 |
| 2. | Number of focus group subjects from each site | 30 |
| 3. | Sequence of questions used to guide focus groups | 30 |
| 4. | Food and nutrition concerns | 33 |
| 5. | Tasks for assessment of functional status | 36 |
| 6. | Structured interview schedule | 40 |
| 7. | Descriptive and analytic outcome variables | 43 |
| 8. | Marital status | 48 |
| 9. | Ethnicity, education, and town of residence | 49 |
| 0. | Age and living situation | 50 |
| 11. | Monthly rent | 50 |
| 12. | Self-reported health and self-reported illness | 52 |
| 13. | Functional status | 53 |
| 14. | Activities of daily living: comparison with national data | 54 |
| 15. | Height, weight, and Body Mass Index | 55 |
| 16. | Body Mass Index values reported in the literature | 57 |
| 17. | Nutrition Screening Initiative DETERMINE checklist scores | 58 |
| 18. | Ranking of nutrition concerns by participants | 75 |
| 19. | Schema of nutrition-related helping behaviors | 76 |
| 20. | Physician- and self-prescribed modified diets | 87 |
| 21. | Diet support providers and types of support | 94 |
| 22. | Satisfaction comparison on diet support | 97 |
| 23. | Incidence of modified diets | 98 |
| 24. | Food and meal procurement support recipients and providers by functional status | 106 |

| | | |
|---|---|---|
| 25. | Food and meal procurement support providers and types of support | 107 |
| 26. | Meal program participation | 108 |
| 27. | Satisfaction comparison on food acquisition support | 111 |
| 28. | Summary of nutrition-related support by source | 114 |
| 29. | Mean nutrient intakes of subjects in comparison to national samples | 122 |
| 30. | Nutrient intakes in comparison to 1989 RDAs | 124 |
| 31. | Calcium intakes, comparison with other groups | 127 |
| 32. | Suggested revisions to the RDAs, compared with intakes | 129 |
| 33. | Diet patterns in comparison to the Dietary Guidelines | 130 |
| 34. | Diet Quality Index | 134 |
| 35. | Dietary scores | 135 |
| 36. | Diet Quality Index, comparison with other groups | 135 |
| 37. | Brief summary of operational definitions of variables | 142 |
| 38. | Hierarchical regression results for functional status, number of helpers and joint relation on DQI | 148 |
| 39. | Simple slope analysis results at each level of functional ability for DQI | 149 |
| 40. | Hierarchical regression results for functional status, number of helpers and joint relation on MAR | 153 |
| 41. | Hierarchical regression results for calories/day, functional status, number of helpers and joint relation on MAR | 157 |
| 42. | Simple slope analysis results at each level of functional ability for MAR, controlled for calories/day | 159 |
| 43. | Hierarchical regression results for functional status, number of types of help and joint relation on diet quality | 160 |
| 44. | Hierarchical regression results for functional status, total helpers + types of help and joint relation on diet quality | 161 |
| 45. | Hierarchical regression results for functional status, satisfaction and joint relation on diet quality | 164 |

# Figures

| | | |
|---|---|---|
| 1. | Proposed model of the association between social relationships and dietary quality | 5 |
| 2. | Distribution on Body Mass Index | 56 |
| 3. | Distribution on social anchorage scores, in comparison to male sample | 61 |
| 4. | Size of diet support network | 89 |
| 5. | Relationship of diet support providers to respondent | 90 |
| 6. | Number of subjects receiving each type of support | 92 |
| 7. | Types of help that subjects feel would benefit their diet effort | 96 |
| 8. | Ascending levels of support in acquiring groceries | 101 |
| 9. | Support in acquiring groceries by functional status | 102 |
| 10. | Support in acquiring meals by functional status | 103 |
| 11. | Relationship of food and meal procurement support providers to respondent | 105 |
| 12. | Average consumption per week of the ten most frequently eaten foods | 118 |
| 13. | Average intake per 1000 calories of the ten highest contributing foods | 119 |
| 14. | Mean Adequacy Ratio | 133 |
| 15. | Proposed model of the association between social relationships and dietary quality | 141 |
| 16. | Graph showing joint relation of functional status and number of helpers on DQI | 151 |
| 17. | Distribution of mean number helpers by functional status | 152 |

18. Average MAR by number of helpers and functional status ... 154
19. Graph showing joint relation of functional status and number of helpers on MAR while controlling for average caloric intake ... 158
20. Distribution of mean number types of help by functional status ... 162

# Acknowledgments

Many individuals have provided encouragement and assistance on this project. My committee members have gently guided me since inception of the research proposal. Dr. Ann Ferris, my major advisor, has been a patient, insightful, and inspirational mentor. I thank her for her confidence in venturing into the complex and unfamiliar realm of social support. I will always appreciate her faith in me and in the success of this project.

I also thank my two associate advisors, Dr. Nancy Rodriguez and Dr. Nancy Sheehan. Dr. Rodriguez was always gracious with practical advice and earnest enthusiasm. Dr. Sheehan broadened my perspective and interpretation of the human situations I attempted to document. My gratitude is also extended to Dr. Jeffery Backstrand for help with proposed statistical analyses, and to Dr. David Kenny for guidance on moderated regression.

I was fortunate to be led by Dr. Sheehan during my Travelers Center on Aging fellowship experience. That opportunity greatly expanded my knowledge of geriatrics and my compassion for older adults. The fellowship training had a significant impact on the research protocol for this study, most importantly on the inclusion of qualitative methods.

I am also indebted to the faculty, staff, and resources of the Department of Nutritional Sciences. Most notably, I am grateful to the personnel and resources of the Senior Nutrition Awareness Program (SNAP). SNAP transformed the project proposal into reality. Moreover, the hard work and pleasant companionship of my fellow interviewers, Diane, Pauline, and Viki considerably brightened the research phase.

Similarly, I thank my fellow graduate students in the department for their camaraderie and technical support. Namanjeet provided my first day tour of the department. Ever since then I have recognized the collaborative spirit of students. I have especially depended on Valerie, Beate, Nancy, Laurie, Linda, Silke, Marcia, Cara, Sandy, and Rebecca.

This project would not have been possible without the help of over 200 benevolent elderly women. I thank these independent females for sharing a glimpse of their personal lives. Likewise, I am grateful to the staff of the housing sites who permitted me to become a part of their community for a brief time.

Finally, I thank my family and friends for their patience, empathy, reassurance, affection, child care and emergency help, and lots of fun times too: my husband, Dennis; my children, Kira, Nolan, and Danika; my parents, Ed and June; and my good friends, Linda, Jody, Karen, Kristine, Thor, Una, Bob, Robin, Polly, Rob, Anneliese, and Anne. Many thanks.

# Nutrition Support to Elderly Women

CHAPTER 1
# Introduction

The growing elderly population suffers from a disproportionately large incidence of chronic and acute illnesses, as well as mental and physical disabilities. The Surgeon General's report on Nutrition and Health points out that "dietary, economic, and social support programs" render significant health benefits to older adults with these chronic conditions (U.S. DHHS 1988). Optimal nutrition speeds recovery from acute illnesses and can help improve or maintain functional status and quality of life (Administration on Aging 1994; Gray-Donald 1995; Palmer 1990; Position of the American Dietetic Association 1996; Rosenberg and Miller 1992).

Supportive relationships can also impact positively on health and quality of life during the later years (Antonucci and Akiyama 1995; Bloom 1990; Broadhead et al. 1983; Grundy, Bowling, and Farquhar 1996). Support from friends and family enhances self-care practices, promotes the use of services, and increases life satisfaction (Hansson and Carpenter 1994). In addition, social support is believed to exert a beneficial effect on food intake (Coe and Miller 1984; Davies and Knutson 1991; Krause and Wray 1991), thereby further increasing the overall influence of social support on health.

The importance of social relationships on the dietary adequacy of elders was recognized at the Nutrition Screening Initiative (NSI) Consensus conference (White 1991). The NSI identified social isolation as one of seven key risk factors predicting nutritional health in older adults. Title IIIC of the Older Americans Act, which mandates nutrition services for the elderly, includes the opportunity for social interaction as an important goal of the program. Congregate meal participants have indicated that the opportunity to socialize is valued (Administration on Aging 1983; Falk, Bisogni, and Sobal 1996; Neyman, Zidenberg-Cherr, and McDonald 1996; Van Zandt 1986).

Thus, public programs incorporate the premise of a positive link between strong social relationships and a high quality diet. However, few research studies have actually been able to document this association. Little is known about the types and attributes of social relationships that influence food patterns. The objective of this study was to explore, in depth, specific aspects of social relationships and their association with dietary quality.

## SOCIAL RELATIONSHIPS

The social network is the set of persons who interact with the focal subject. Typically, network structure is defined in terms of nodes (people) and ties (bonds between nodes) (Antonucci 1985). Structural identifiers, such as size, stability, homogeneity, complexity, and density are used to distinguish properties of the network.

The social network may contain both informal (kin, friends, neighbors) and formal (professional, government) sources. Both provide various functions that impact on the physical and mental status of the focal subject. By integrating the literature from research on social isolation, loneliness, and social support, Rook (1985) has suggested a schema for conceptualizing the functions of social bonds.[1] Her interpretation is useful in understanding the influence of social relationships on food intake patterns.

Rook (1985) proposes three functions of social bonds: companionship, social control, and social support. Companionship provides intimacy and pleasure. The primary function of companionship is to increase feelings of self-worth and self-esteem. Social control exerts a regulatory function. Social ties inhibit deviant behavior while promoting healthful habits, especially during transitional periods. Social support operates during times of need. Tangible aid, information, or emotional support may be extended to offset debilitating effects of a stressful event.

Figure 1: Proposed model of the association between social relationships and dietary quality (adapted from Rook 1985)

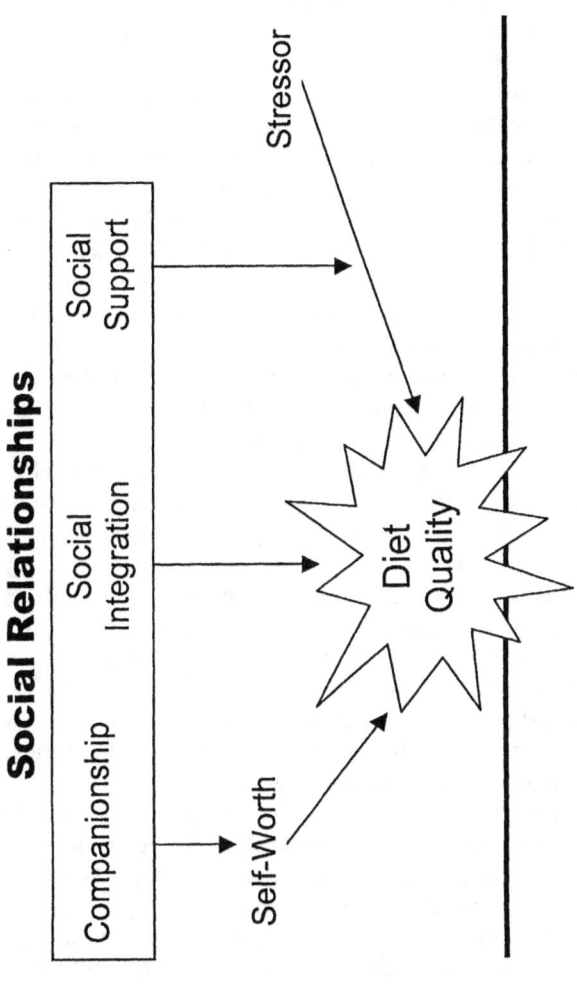

In Figure 1, a nutrition-specific adaptation of Rook's model is proposed. Rook explains that the presence of a companion increases feelings of self-worth. Heightened self-worth leads to mental well being, happiness, and life satisfaction. In the nutrition-specific model, the increase in self-worth has a beneficial impact on dietary quality (Coe and Miller 1984; Schafer, Keith, and Schafer 1994). The influence of companionship on diet quality is therefore indirect, operating through self-worth.

The second function of social relationships, social control, is presented as social integration in Figure 1. Social integration is the degree to which the focal individual feels a part of the community. The more socially integrated, the more control society would be expected to exert. The alternative is social isolation. A gradual withdrawal from social activities often occurs during the later years (Sauer and Coward 1985). Rook proposes that the subsequent social isolation could provoke role ambivalence and inadequate self-care behaviors. For instance, a socially withdrawn individual may choose to eat cold cereal three times a day and not experience the normative guilt of such a deed. Thus, in the nutrition-specific model, social integration would have a direct and consistent effect on diet quality.

In contrast, social support, the third function of social relationships, is only activated in response to a stressful occurrence in the life of the focal subject. The goal of support providers is to help the focal individual through a short- or long-term period of difficulty. In the nutrition-specific model, social support moderates the influence of a potential nutrition-related stressor. For example, a newly diagnosed diabetic must change her eating patterns to follow an explicit, prescribed diet. Without diet instruction or encouragement, she is likely to have poor dietary compliance and a poor prognosis. However, with optimal support from health professionals, family, and friends, she can control her diabetes with a high quality diet.

In summary, social relationships are postulated to affect diet quality through indirect (companionship), direct (integration), and interactive (support) modes. Unfortunately, prior studies investigating social relationships and diet quality have not always employed similar definitions. For instance, structural measures of social integration have been included most frequently, but have been labeled as indices of social support. Furthermore, some prior indices simultaneously assess more than one function. The following discussion of research findings shows how multiple definitions of the social relationship construct have led to uncertain conclusions.

The literature search was limited to research involving older adults. Both foodways (Hendricks, Calasanti, and Turner 1988) and social relationships (Antonucci 1985) vary with age. Although the category of older adults contains a very heterogeneous mix, inclusion of younger individuals would have compelled even greater variability.

## PRIOR RESEARCH

Although nutrition researchers have endeavored to investigate the influence of social relationships on diet quality in the elderly, the proxy measures most often employed have not been adequate to address the complexity of the constructs. The following discussion first describes research efforts that have included a nonspecific measure of social relationships. The results of research employing indices that can be categorized according to the adapted model are then described.

### Living Arrangement

Most frequently, an assessment of social bonds has been included in studies examining multiple psychosocial factors. Thus researchers have needed a simple measure to represent the complex phenomena of social relationships. The most typical proxy measure is the living arrangement of the older adult, that is, whether the elder lives alone or with others. Living alone is believed to increase vulnerability to inadequate social interaction, a lack of companionship, and insufficient social support (Rubinstein, Lubben, and Mintzer 1994; White 1991). In other words, living alone is expected to negatively impact all three of the functions of social relationships in the proposed model.

Some studies have documented that older adults who live alone consume a less nutritious diet than individuals who live with others (Bianchetti et al. 1990; Reid and Miles 1977; Slesinger, McDivitt, and O'Donnell 1980). However, most researchers have found no relationship (Kolasa, Mitchell, and Jobe 1995; LeClerc and Thornbury 1983; Payette et al. 1995; Posner, Smigelski, and Krachenfels 1987; Ryan and Bower 1989; Sem et al. 1988; Zipp and Holcomb 1992).

Davis et al. conducted detailed analyses of National Health and Examination Survey 1971 to 1974 (NHANES I) and Nationwide Food Consumption Survey 1977 to 1978 (NFCS) data (Davis et al. 1985 and 1990, respectively). The results of both surveys indicate that older males who live alone have the poorest diets. The diet quality of older females who live alone is equivalent to the diet quality of older adults who live with others. Similarly, Frongillo et al. (1992) and Westenbrink et al. (1989) found that the combination of male gender and living alone appears to increase risk of a deficient diet.

Horwath (1989) suggests that gender and living arrangement are indicators of larger social forces. In this elderly cohort, females have been the traditional providers of food and nutrition. Simultaneously, females have shouldered the responsibilities of maintaining social networks. The poor diet quality of elderly men who live alone may result from limited knowledge of food procurement and preparation methods. An inadequate support network may further exacerbate the situation.

In summary, the results of research examining the association between living arrangement and diet quality suggest that living alone may have a slight, negative impact on food intake patterns, especially for males. In other words, for certain groups of older adults, inadequate opportunities for socialization may inhibit healthy eating behaviors. This conclusion is further supported by research of Hubbard, Muhlenkamp, and Brown (1984). Their assessment of the interpersonal resources of older adults tapped all three functions of social relationships. Elders with strong social resources employed more positive health behaviors, including good nutrition practices, than elders with low social resources.

**Companionship**

According to Rook (1985), companionship includes both pleasurable camaraderie and emotional sharing. Pleasurable camaraderie refers to joint recreation and leisure time activities. Emotional sharing is typified by confidential discussions of personal feelings. The results of these activities are enhanced mood and increased self-worth. Mutually shared affection also results in decreased loneliness, increased happiness, and greater life satisfaction (Rook 1985).

Only two research studies have examined the relationship between companionship and diet quality in the elderly. Hanson, Mattisson, and Steen (1987) assessed perceived availability and adequacy of emotionally close relationships in 480 males, age 68. Analyses of diet history data revealed that 20% of the men had diets of poor quality, specified as one or more nutrients below a defined cut-off. Chi-square results indicated no statistically significant association between diet quality and level of perceived closeness. However, a trend was apparent in the expected direction. Men with poorer diets did report lower relationship availability and adequacy ratings than men with good diets. The data categorization methods and use of chi-square may have weakened the ability to detect statistically significant associations (Blalock 1979).

In the second study examining companionship and diet quality, Heller and Mansbach (1984) assessed three aspects of close relationships. Forty-three elderly women reported the number of intimates in their network, the proportion of intimates to total network, and the frequency of contact with intimates. No association with the intake of four nutrients was found. The researchers attributed the lack of significance to the small sample size and the limitations of a 24-hour recall to determine diet adequacy.

Referring to the nutrition-specific model, the proposed association between companionship and diet quality is indirect. In support of the model, Heller and Mansbach (1984) did find that the proportion of intimates to total network entered into a predictive multiple regression equation for life satisfaction. However, in their sample, life satisfaction was not related to the intake of any of the four nutrients.

Only a limited number of research studies have explored the pathway from self-concept to diet quality (Witte, Skinner, and Carruth 1991). Schafer and Keith (1982) noted no relationship between self-esteem and diet in their sample of single and married older adults. In contrast, Learner and Kivett (1981) found that elders who perceived problems with their diet also reported lower morale. The researchers credited the low morale to loneliness. The findings of Walker and Beauchene (1991) are in agreement with this proposition. Participants in their study completed the UCLA Loneliness Questionnaire and three days of diet records. Loneliness was associated with poorer nutrient intakes.

In conclusion, the nutrition-specific model suggests that companionship influences diet through the effect on self-worth. Only two studies were found which examined a direct relationship between companionship and diet quality in older adults. Neither study found a significant association. Furthermore, only four projects have considered the link between attributes of self-concept and diet. Results are inconclusive. Of the three dimensions of social relationships, the influence of companionship on diet quality appears the least well understood. Future studies are needed in this area.

**Social Integration**

Rook (1985) posits social integration as the second function of relationships. The unique contribution of integration lies in the regulation of behavior. Individuals who are socially embedded are more likely to follow cultural norms. Social roles and obligations provide guidelines for appropriate behaviors. The input of others deters socially integrated individuals from deviant conduct and encourages healthful activities, such as good nutritional habits.

One dimension of social integration is membership in a family. The role of spouse or parent carries certain responsibilities, but does not always indicate emotional closeness (Seeman and Berkman 1988). In a sample of 314 married older adults, Mullins and Mushel (1992) found that 51% did not feel emotionally close to their spouse. Of 757 who were parents, 40% were not close to any of their children.

Regardless, the socially defined roles and responsibilities as spouse or parent may still be expected to encourage self-care practices. However, studies examining these attributes have not consistently shown a relationship to eating patterns. McIntosh, Shifflett, and Picou (1989) found that married individuals had better intakes of vitamin/minerals, protein, and calories than did unmarried persons. Other researchers have found no relationship between marital status and diet quality (Hunter and Linn 1979; Sem et al. 1988). Sem et al. did note more "always single" elderly in the group with the lowest diet score. In contrast, Schafer and Keith (1982) found that elderly, single females had better diets than married couples.

Davis et al. (1985) simultaneously considered marital status and gender. They reported that males who lived with a spouse had better diets than males who lived with others. Marital status had no association to diet quality in females. Number of children (Cohen and Ralston 1992; Payette et al. 1995) and closeness to children (Cohen and Ralston 1992) have been found to be unrelated to nutrient intakes.

A somewhat related measure of social integration is mealtime companionship. Eating is considered a social activity. Furthermore, elders often engage in food activities simply because they offer an opportunity to socialize (Falk, Bisogni, and Sobal 1996). One informant of Howarth (1993, 74–75) reported:

> "I should say I lost my husband three years ago. And he (the neighbor) used to have his meals with us for years and years and years and he still has them with me. So he's kind of more than my neighbor he's like a younger brother . . ."

Sharing food appears to influence the level of social companionship.

Some researchers have hypothesized that the reverse also holds — that mealtime companionship influences the level of nutritional quality. Eating with others does appear to improve appetite and increase the amount of food which is consumed (de Castro 1994).

However, researchers have not found that mealtime companionship improves the quality of the diet (Cohen and Ralston 1992; LeClerc and Thornbury 1983; Payette et al. 1995), nor the perception of diet problems (Learner and Kivett 1981). Using the same data set as Learner and Kivett, Kinard and Kivett (1983) reported that mealtime companionship was not related to morale. The lack of a relationship between mealtime companionship and morale supports the use of this variable as a proxy for social integration rather than companionship. The overall conclusion is that while eating with others may increase the quantity of food that is consumed, mealtime companionship does not appear to increase the nutritional quality of the food.

In nutrition research, the most frequent indicator of social interaction is a measure of social contacts. The frequency of contact with friends and relatives has shown no association with diet quality in numerous studies (Coe and Miller 1984; Cohen and Ralston 1992; Hanson, Mattisson, and Steen 1987; Heller and Mansbach 1984; Payette et al. 1995; Sem et al. 1988; Walker and Beauchene 1991; Zipp and Holcomb 1992). Only two documented a positive association

(Clancy 1975; McIntosh and Shifflett 1984). Furthermore, network size, density (Cohen and Ralston 1992; Heller and Mansbach 1984), proximity, church membership (Cohen and Ralston 1992), and participation in the community (Hanson, Mattisson, and Steen 1987) have not shown relationships with dietary adequacy.

In summary, all of the social integration measures discussed thus far show little, if any, relationship to diet quality. Marital status, number of children, mealtime companionship, and frequency of contact all assess structural attributes of the network. The purpose of the interactions and the quality of the interactions may be more important than the quantity. The functions of social relationships, rather than network attributes, have more frequently shown an association with other health behaviors and outcomes (Hendricks and Calasanti 1986; Kriegsman, Penninx, and van Eijk 1995; Pearlin et al. 1981). Furthermore, network properties are not reliable indicators of social functions (Cutrona 1986; Revicki and Mitchell 1986; Rubinstein, Lubben, and Mintzer 1994; Seeman and Berkman 1988).

In agreement with this argument, studies that assessed satisfaction with frequency of contact found an association with perceived diet problems (Learner and Kivett 1981) and nutritional risk (Coe et al. 1984). These results indicate that the association depends on the quality rather than the quantity of contact (Chappell and Badger 1989). Further support is found in the results by Hanson, Mattisson, and Steen (1987) in their previously discussed study of 68-year-old men. These researchers reported an association between social anchorage, or a sense of belonging in the community, and dietary adequacy. In addition, social anchorage was inversely related to BMI. That is, a low *feeling of* belonging was related to a poor nutrient intake and a high BMI.

In conclusion, the few studies assessing the perceived quality of social integration are in accordance. Feeling socially embedded has a positive effect on the quality of the diet. However, structural network indicators demonstrate only a limited association with diet. The quantity of social interaction does not appear to significantly influence *the quality* of food patterns.

## Social Support

The third function of social relationships is support during times of stress (Rook 1985). Social support includes emotional, informational, and instrumental types of help extended in response to an identified need (Hansson and Carpenter 1994). **Emotional support** promotes a positive attitude. Examples include expressions of encouragement, understanding, and reassurance. **Informational support** refers to shared knowledge, for instance providing literature or suggestions on how to resolve the problem. **Instrumental support** consists of material and tangible types of aid, such as transportation, labor, or financial help.

All three types of support may be offered in response to one problem. Consider the example of an elderly woman with deteriorating vision. She has recently relinquished her driving license and is feeling a disheartening loss of independence. In response to her distress, network members offer support. Instrumental support might include offers to drive her to activities and appointments. Informational types of support might include bus schedules and introduction to the Senior Van. Emotional support might include affirmation of worth, regardless of driving ability, and empathetic listening to her lamentations.

Emotional support differs from the emotional exchanges of companionship because of purpose (Rook 1985). In the above example, affirming the worth of the elder was a response to the stressful circumstances. In another situation, a candle-lit dinner for instance, affirming worth might be an expression of emotional intimacy. In Rook's model, supportive exchanges serve to bring a stressed individual back to a prior level of function, or well being. In contrast, companionship heightens feelings of self-worth.

Rook also limits the category of supportive behaviors to affirming, positive interactions. Network members may also use derogatory intervention methods, such as hiding the car keys prior to an individual's giving up her license. These types of actions are classified under the function of social integration.

Social support therefore, refers to positive actions initiated by members of the network. The actions are offered in response to a stressful occurrence in the life of the focal individual. In general, emotional, instrumental, or informational types of help may be offered.

Three studies have examined the direct association between social support and diet quality. Two of the studies have been previously discussed: the study of 480 68–year-old men by Hanson, Mattisson, and Steen (1987) and the sample of 43 elderly women by Heller and Mansbach (1984). Neither of these researchers found a relationship between their measure of perceived social support and diet quality.

Hanson, Mattisson, and Steen (1987) assessed the availability of material and informational support in the community. The scale consisted of five items. One point was awarded for each item if the participant knew someone who could provide that type of help. Thus the scores ranged from one to five. The scale was then broken into low, medium, and high groupings for chi-square analyses. The dependent variable was a poor diet, defined as having one or more nutrients below a specified cut-off.

As in the results for emotional closeness previously discussed, the difference between groups was not statistically significant (p=.17). However, the same trend was apparent. Men with poor diets were more likely to perceive low levels of support. Again, the categorization necessary for chi-square analysis may have limited the power of the analyses.

Furthermore, 80% of Hanson's participants were married. The instrument to assess social support was designed to minimize support from the wife. However, wives are often the sole source of support for married men (Kriegsman, Penninx, and van Eijk 1995). Ignoring spousal contributions may obscure important differences that exist between men with supportive wives, men with unsupportive wives, and men without wives. In addition, wives often have more influence on food patterns than do their husbands. Analysis of the interaction between the support variable and marital status might have revealed some interesting associations.

The research of Heller and Mansbach (1984) used an alternative measure of support. Subjects first listed up to ten people in their social network. For each network member, the subject then reported:

1. if the network member might provide emotional support in response to a problem situation, and
2. if the network member might provide instrumental support in response to a problem.

## Introduction

The total amount of each type of support was then summed and divided by the size of the network. Two average support scores were thus derived for each subject. The intakes of four nutrients from a 24-hour recall (protein, iron, vitamin A, and vitamin D) were the diet outcome measures. No relationships between support and diet were found.

Both the dependent and independent measures have limitations in this study. The support instrument assumes that the average level of support is the essential element. Thus an individual who received support from her only two network members would receive a higher score (score = 1) than a second individual who received support from four out of her eight network members (score = 0.5). As for the dependent variable, a 24-hour recall is insufficient to derive nutrient intake scores. Furthermore, the researchers noted little diet variability in their subjects. All the women ate one meal of the day at the congregate meal site from which they were recruited.

The third study examining the direct relationship between social support and diet quality was conducted by Toner (1987; Toner and Morris 1992). Toner created a Nutrition Support Questionnaire, based on the Inventory of Socially Supportive Behaviors (ISSB—of Barrera, Sandler, and Ramsay 1981; subsequently modified by Krause 1989). Participants indicated how often they had received 14 different types of support from health professionals and from family, friends, and neighbors. In addition, subjects reported how often they had provided these types of support to others. An example of one question is, *"Check how often someone has discussed with you how to prepare or select nutritious foods."*

A 24-hour recall was used to determine food intake. Nutrient adequacy ratios were calculated for 13 vitamins and minerals plus protein. Support from family, friends, and neighbors was associated with the intake of five of nineteen nutrients and a summary score ($r=.19$ to $.28$, $p<.05$). No correlation existed between support from formal sources nor with support given to others (reciprocal support) and nutrient intakes.

The use of a 24-hour recall is a limitation of Toner's study, as in Heller and Mansbach. Additionally, her statistical analyses consisted of multiple correlations between each nutrient and the three dimensions of social support (plus two dimensions of self-actualization plus further variables, not discussed here). A statistical adjustment, such as the Bonferroni procedure, should have been employed to decrease Type I error (Pedhazur 1997). The inflated error due to these two factors leaves little confidence in the results.

Furthermore, Toner's support scale assessed enacted support. The questions asked about types of help that had already been received. *"Check how often someone has helped you with food preparation."* Yet Toner did not assess the degree of need. A fully functional older adult would not need help with food preparation. Thus, the amount of help that a fully functional older adult received in this area would not be expected to affect diet quality.

Rook (1985) emphasizes that social support is offered during times of need. A stressor must be present in order for the support network to be mobilized. To adequately assess the influence of social support on diet, both the level of stress and the level of social support must be considered. Only one study was found that analyzed the statistical interaction of social relationships and a stressor on diet in an elderly sample (McIntosh, Shifflett, and Picou 1989).

Unfortunately, the project of McIntosh, Shifflett, and Picou (1989) is a secondary analysis of a data set not originally intended to examine social support and stress. The sample consisted of 170 elderly persons with a mean age of 69 years. The researchers employed principal components factor analyses (PCA) to form composite indicator variables.

Two social relationship factors were derived:

- friendship network: "number of close friends, friendship density, frequency of getting together with close friends, and the extent to which advice was shared with friends," and
- companionship: "mealtime companionship, and help with cooking."

Friendship network incorporates attributes of all three dimensions of Rook's model, but seems to lean most towards social integration. Companionship is also difficult to categorize, containing both social integration and support components. PCA was also used to identify:

- financial stress: the ability to pay for food, clothes, and medicine,
- appetite: three statements describing appetite, and
- vitamin/mineral: composite of 9 vitamins and minerals.

Multiple regression was used to investigate the direct and interactive effects on appetite. Marital status was statistically controlled in all equations. In the additive (direct) model, companionship was not related to appetite. Extended friendship network was related to a better appetite. Financial strain decreased appetite.

In the interactive model, the interaction of friendship network and financial stress on appetite was statistically significant. An extensive friendship network buffered against the potentially detrimental effects of financial stress on appetite. The interaction of companionship and financial stress was also significant, but in the opposite direction. Companionship evidently increased the depressant effects of financial strain on appetite. In turn, appetite was related to vitamin/mineral and protein intakes.

The results are difficult to interpret. Statistically, the interactive model was preferable, accounting for 37% of the variance. The additive model only accounted for 14%. McIntosh, Shifflett, and Picou (1989) concluded that friends are more beneficial than family in buffering individuals from the negative impacts of financial strain on appetite. They hypothesized that the help with cooking indicated a loss of control, thus the depressant effect on appetite.

The results clearly illustrate the need for more research. Interesting joint effects of financial stress and social relationships on appetite were apparent that warrant further study. The tentative model of McIntosh, Shifflett, and Picou (1989) was insightful, but the results are difficult to interpret due to the data set and reliance on PCA factors. In contrast, Toner's (1987) assessment of nutrition support was more thorough, but she lacked a comprehensive model. Her results would have been more informative had she simultaneously considered level of nutrition-related stress.

**Summary of Research Findings**

In summary, Rook (1985) has integrated the findings from research in the areas of social isolation, loneliness, and social support. She offers a consolidated view of the association between social relationships and well being. Based on her perspective, a nutrition-specific model has been proposed to describe the influence of social relationships on diet quality.

The three functions of social relationships include companionship, social integration, and social support. The majority of prior nutrition studies examining social relationships have assessed a composite of all three functions or have examined aspects of social integration. Most researchers have investigated structural network properties, such as living situation, marital status, and frequency of contact with friends and relatives. Overall the results suggest that some type of positive link exists between social relationships and diet quality. However, the association appears weak. The structural network indicators are unable to proxy for the substance and character of social relationships.

Few nutrition studies have assessed the more qualitative indicators of social relationships, such as availability of a confident, social embeddedness, or types of support. Furthermore, most of these have only considered the direct association between social relationships and diet, overlooking buffering effects and indirect influences. Moreover, inadequate controls have been placed on related variables, such as gender and special diet needs.

All three functions of social relationships are likely to impact on the diet quality of older adults. Companionship, integration, and support all have the potential to encourage self-care practices, but the situations and modes of operation differ. This research study focuses specifically on the relationship between social support and diet quality. Thus stress must also be considered; the entity that sets social support in motion. An investigation of social support must simultaneously investigate stress.

## STRESS

Stress is a condition or occurrence that threatens well being (Pearlin 1989). Types of stress are often categorized as daily hassles, life events, or chronic stressors (Chiriboga 1989; George 1989; Pearlin 1989).

# Introduction

Daily hassles are the minor irritants of everyday life. For example, sleeping through the alarm and getting a late start on the day, finding that the milk carton is empty *after* pouring the bowl of cereal, and realizing that the shirt you had planned to wear is still in the wash. Life events include identifiable changes in life patterns, such as death of a relative, purchase of a house, and starting a new job. Chronic stressors are enduring, burdensome conditions. Examples include chronic illness, role responsibility overload, and poverty. Older adults also appear stressed by future events and nonexperienced events (Linn 1986) as well as difficult circumstances of their children and friends (Chiriboga 1989).

Each of these types of stress impacts on physical and mental health. The degree of impact depends on the perceptions and expectations of the stressed person (Pearlin 1989). Nonnormative and unplanned occurrences appear the most detrimental to health. However, the negative effects of daily hassles can be just as severe as the negative impacts of life events (Chiriboga 1989). In part, the similar outcomes result from the contagious nature of stressors. Individuals who are exposed to one stress are likely to be exposed to additional stresses at all levels. Pearlin (1989) suggests that an identified stressor is merely an indicator of more general social disorganization in the life of an individual.

Because food consumption is essential for health, and an everyday event, many types of stress have the potential to affect nutritional intake. **Daily hassles** such as running out of milk or skipping breakfast to avoid being late for work are obvious examples that alter food intake patterns. Less obvious is the way that minor irritations may build during the day to finally impact on the dinner meal, either in the choice of foods or in the atmosphere at the table.

**Life events** may also alter eating habits. Widowhood is one illustration. Individuals recently widowed report a reduced appetite and derangement of meal patterns (Rosenbloom and Whittington 1993). Financial difficulties provide another instance. Food is often the expense category that must be compromised. Housing and utilities are relatively inelastic. The greater the number of recent life events, the larger the expected impact on diet quality. One research study found that the greater the number of stressful life events the lower the protein intake in 145 elderly subjects (Payette et al. 1995).

Of relevance is that "a change in food habits" is one of the most frequent life event stressors reported by older adults (Chiriboga 1989; Linn 1986). Kolasa, Mitchell, and Jobe (1995) found that 44% of their random sample of 2178 older adults reported a change in food habits within the past five years. The life event scales do not inquire about the cause of the change. Other life events may frequently be the basis, illustrating the concept of aggregation of stressors. Widowhood, illness, or relocation are just a few of the simultaneous stressors that might trigger a change in eating habits.

**Chronic stress** may also impinge on eating patterns. A chronic stressor that appears particularly salient to food intake patterns of the elderly is a loss in the ability to perform typical activities of daily living (Administration on Aging 1994). Often termed functional status, the ability to perform self-care and home management skills may be temporarily or permanently impaired due to physical or mental disabilities. Functional abilities often are categorized as "basic activities of daily living" (BADL) such as dressing, grooming, walking, and bathing; and "instrumental activities of daily living" (IADL) such as shopping, using the telephone, and cleaning the house. Environmental and social adaptations can permit a return to previous lifestyle patterns regardless of functional impairments.

Frongillo et al. (1992) reported that bed- and chair-bound recipients of home delivered meals were more likely than more mobile recipients to skip all meals for at least one day. Older adults with greater IADL limitations were more likely to have changed their eating habits than individuals with fewer limitations in the large random sample of Kolasa et al. (1995). These findings suggest that functional limitations result in altered food intakes.

Low, but significant relationships between functional status and diet quality ($r=.21$ to $.28$) have been reported (Hunter and Linn 1979; Walker and Beauchene 1991). That is, individuals with more functional impairments consume less adequate diets. Bianchetti et al. (1990) demonstrated that the loss of only one or more IADL skills was enough to signify a poorer nutrient intake in 1303 elderly persons. Using multiple regression, Betts and Vivian (1985) noted that BADL/IADL ability in 100 older adults affected dietary adequacy to a greater extent than social resources, physical health, mental health, or economic resources, as assessed by the OARS Multidimensional Functional Assessment Instrument.

Furthermore, impaired functional status was associated with high BMI, an indicator of nutritional status, in participants of the Longitudinal Study on Aging (LSOA) (Harris et al. 1989). Galanos et al. (1994) found a curvilinear relationship existed in the NHANES I sample. Poor functional status was related to BMIs below the 5$^{th}$ percentile and above the 85$^{th}$ percentile. The curvilinear relationship may have been missed in the LSOA group since the researchers categorized by quartiles.

In summary, a reduced ability to perform typical, daily activities has been associated with a change in eating habits, diet of poorer quality, and undesirable BMI. However, family, friends, neighbors and social service agencies are likely to extend support when functional status declines. The perception of a supportive network as well as the actual provision of emotional, informational, and tangible aid may alter the older adult's appraisal of the situation (Cohen and Wills 1985). Coping abilities are enhanced and the negative influences on eating patterns may be reduced when social support is available. The relationship between functional capabilities and diet quality is therefore more complex and perhaps even more salient than noted in previous research.

## CONCLUSION

Older adults require an adequate diet to optimize health and quality of life. A feeling of social integration, and perhaps the availability of a confidant, appears to positively influence elderly persons towards more healthful eating behaviors. However, stressful situations may arise which disrupt normal patterns. A diminished ability to perform self-care skills is one stressor that negatively affects diet quality. Fortunately, social support may be mobilized in response to the decline in functional status. Support has the potential to buffer against detrimental effects on diet. The impact on food intake most likely depends on the level of functional impairment as well as the quality of the social support system.

Further research is needed to more fully understand the ability of social support to mediate the effects of impaired functional status on diet quality. Different types of aid offered by the social network and different role relationships may vary in their effects. Moreover, negative perceptions of support may also arise, which have yet to be investigated in conjunction with dietary intake. Finally, additional measures of nutritional status, such as physiological indices, need to be examined.

## OBJECTIVES

Because prior research has not focused on nutrition-specific social support, the first goal of this study was to explore and describe the current situation in a group of elderly women living alone in government subsidized housing. Who are the providers of nutrition-related support? What types of support are they offering? How satisfied are the recipients with the support? The second goal was to examine the relationships between nutrition-related support, a stressor, and diet quality according to the adapted Rook model. Thus, both descriptive outcomes and analytic hypotheses were proposed for this study. The specific objectives are stated below.

### Descriptive outcomes

1. A classification scheme of nutrition-related helping behaviors, as reported by older women, will be developed.
2. The frequency of instrumental, informational, and emotional social support functions will be examined in response to identified food and nutrition problems of elders. In addition, the providers of the various types of support will be identified.
3. The older women's satisfaction with nutrition-related social support will be described. Again, the providers of the support will be considered simultaneously.

### Analytic research hypotheses

1. Impaired functional status will have a negative effect on diet quality.
2. Enacted, nutrition-related social support will mitigate the effects of impaired functional status on diet quality.

*Introduction* 23

3. Similarly, satisfaction with nutrition-related social support (regardless of the actual level of support) will mitigate the effects of impaired functional status on diet quality.

## OVERVIEW OF BOOK

The following chapters contain a description of the methods and findings of the research project designed to meet the aforementioned objectives. In the next chapter, the methods are described in detail. The research progression can be divided into two phases. Phase I consisted of qualitative methods exploring nutrition problems and related types of support. Phase II involved structured interviews with a larger sample based on the findings of the first phase.

The presentation of findings begins in Chapter 3 with a description of the subjects. Chapter 4 presents a detailed explanation of the Phase I qualitative results, including a categorization scheme of nutrition-related helping behaviors. As the methods of the second phase were based on this categorization scheme, all subsequent chapters build on these findings.

Chapter 5 provides the frequency of providers and functions of social support reported by subjects in the second research phase. Chapter 6 describes the results of a food frequency analysis. Finally, in Chapter 7 the relationship between nutrition-related social support and diet quality is discussed. Chapter 8 contains the conclusions and recommendations for future research in this area.

The findings in Chapter 3 and all subsequent chapters are discussed in comparison to relevant information reported in existing literature. Thus, this monograph presents findings and their implications concurrently within each chapter.

## NOTES

1. Many models of social relationships exist. Conceptualizations of social support in particular are quite heterogeneous (Barrera 1986). For instance, some researchers include companionship as a type of social support, rather than as a separate category of relationship (Antonucci 1985; Vaux 1988). Other theorists do not exclude potential sources of negative support (Wellman and Wortley 1989). Yet others contend that support operates even in the absence of a stressor (Thoits 1982). Furthermore, support can be characterized as enacted

(received), perceived (available if needed), reciprocal (give and take), or acceptable (level of satisfaction). Each framework has strengths and limitations. Rook's interpretation appears promising for this nutrition based study. However, different dimensions of the support construct are relevant for different outcomes (George 1989). Future nutrition research within alternative frameworks would provide additional insights.

CHAPTER 2
# Methods

The goal of this study was to examine the providers and types of nutrition-related social support as perceived by elderly women. The review of literature and early pilot work demonstrated the need to simultaneously assess level of stress with level of support. First, focus groups were held to explore the types of problems that elderly women believe have a negative impact on their eating patterns. Key informant interviews were then conducted to learn the types of helping behaviors offered in response to the identified problems. Ultimately, a larger sample was interviewed to determine the frequency of support and the relationship between support and diet quality. The progression of the research project is summarized in Table 1.

This research was partially funded by the Storrs Agricultural Experiment Station and the University of Connecticut Family Nutrition Program (FNP).

## PILOT STUDIES

As demonstrated in the review of literature, little prior research has focused on the functions of nutrition-specific social support. Early pilot work for this study began in the summer of 1992 to explore types and providers of nutrition help. First, unstructured interviews (Weiss 1994) were held with 15 older females, singly or in small groups. The women discussed the types of problems they experience that they feel have a negative impact on their food intakes.

**Table 1: Progression of research**

I. Phase I: Qualitative Assessment
   A. Four focus groups (n=35)
      1. Moderator led
      2. Audio tape-based content analysis
      3. Confirmatory follow-up interviews (n=5)
      4. Outcome: List of relevant nutrition concerns
   B. Key informant interviews (n=12)
      1. In-depth, open-ended interviews
      2. Audio tape-based content analysis
      3. Outcome: Schema of nutrition-related helping behaviors
II. Phase II: Quantitative Data Collection
   A. Structured interviews (n=102)
      1. Two to three session, comprehensive interviews
      2. Statistical analysis
         i. Independent variables = Social support and Functional status
         ii. Dependent variable = Diet quality
      3. Outcome: Descriptive data and statistical measures of association

Five additional elderly women then participated in in-depth interviews about members of their support networks. The convoy approach of Kahn and Antonucci (1981) was employed. This approach encourages detailed understanding of the relative importance of relationships, the ties between relationships, and the functions of the relationships.

Each of the five respondents described the providers and types of help activated in response to specific nutrition problems. The respondents were also asked to imagine how they would handle additional problems that might happen in the future. Potential providers and types of support were discussed. Common themes were extracted from the notes related to the nutrition problems and the response of social support network members. The enacted, or actual, types and providers of current support appeared more related to present eating patterns than perceived or future support.

Based on these results a structured support questionnaire was developed to assess enacted types and providers of nutrition help. The instrument followed the format of Krause's support scale. (Krause's scale is a modification of the Inventory of Socially Supportive Behaviors by Barrera, Sandler, and Ramsay 1981, [Krause and

Markides 1990]). An example of one question is *"In the past year has anyone brought you groceries?"*

Sixty independently living women, age 65 to 95 years, who were participating in an olfactory study completed the support instrument. The questionnaire also served as a springboard for further unstructured, exploratory interviewing regarding nutrition-related support networks. In general, the respondents were high functioning with few health problems. (These women were not involved in any later phases of this research.)

Only a small number of the women reported the receipt of instrumental or emotional types of nutrition assistance. More of the respondents acknowledged informational aid. The respondents who had not received any support found the questions regarding satisfaction with support difficult to answer. Furthermore, the results of the questionnaire were difficult to interpret since nutrition problems were not simultaneously assessed. For instance, not having a confidant who *"listened to your concerns regarding your diet"* would only indicate inadequate support for a respondent with diet concerns.

The results of the pilot work demonstrated that an investigation of nutrition-related social support needs to assess both the level of perceived nutrition problems and the subsequent enacted support. Researchers focusing on physical and mental health models have noted previously that the functions and providers of social support are specific to the situation (Cohen and Wills 1985; Pearlin et al. 1981). The pilot results suggested that a specific and synergistic relationship exists between stress and support in a nutrition situation as well.

## SUBJECT SELECTION

Nonexperimental research is often the only method to accurately study behavior as it naturally occurs in complex, real-world situations (Pedhazur 1997). However, the researcher must follow a careful design, based on theory, to verify the presence or absence of relationships between variables. In this project, strict subject selection criteria were established to control influences on social support and diet quality.

Potential respondents were recruited from government subsidized housing complexes. Selection criteria included:

- female,
- age 75 to 95,
- lived alone a minimum of five years,
- lived in present location a minimum of two years, and
- sound mental functioning.

Previous researchers have noted that opportunistic samples are likely to be in better health than the sample they represent (Smiciklas-Wright et al. 1990). This study focused on functional status. Thus, the functional abilities of the sample needed to be well distributed. Consequently, recruitment efforts encouraged participation by frail elders. Furthermore, potential recruits with IADL or BADL disabilities were disproportionally selected.

The selection criteria were chosen to control nonstudy variables as well. For instance, gender has been noted to have a significant impact on both diet quality (Hunter and Linn 1979; O'Hanlon et al. 1983) and social network systems (Antonucci and Akiyama 1995; Seelbach 1978). A female sample was designated for this study since the majority of persons in the specified age category are women (Kinsella 1995). Residents in government subsidized housing were recruited to control socioeconomic status and subsequent influence on dietary patterns and social support (Administration on Aging 1994; Krause and Borawski-Clark 1995; Ryan and Bower 1989). In addition, the use of government subsidized apartments controlled for the availability of proximally close age-peer neighbors. Recent widowhood (Rosenbloom and Whittington 1993) and relocation (Wolf 1994) are stressors that may alter food behaviors and social network structure, thus the time criteria for inclusion in the study. The age range 75 to 95 years was selected to restrict cohort effects while permitting a reasonable sample size to be obtained.

Focus group participants were thanked with a gift basket raffle after the discussion. Focus group follow-up participants and key informants were given a $5.00 honorarium. Phase II participants were given a $10.00 honorarium. The procedures were explained to each potential subject before the interviews began and written consent was obtained. The University of Connecticut Human Subjects Review Committee approved procedures.

## PHASE I: FOCUS GROUPS AND KEY INFORMANT INTERVIEWS

Qualitative data were collected and analyzed in the first phase to discern the perceptions and specific situations of women in the identified population. All procedures of Phase I were carried out in cooperation with the Connecticut Housing and Finance Authority (CHFA).

### Focus Groups

Nutrition researchers have identified multiple dietary problems of elderly persons. However, the perceptions of older adults may differ. To ascertain their concerns, four focus groups were held in the winter and spring of 1995. Focus groups are an effective method of generating the spectrum of concerns. The group situation encourages the production of ideas (Morgan 1988; Vaughn, Schumm, and Sinagub 1996). In addition, perceived problems are couched in the language of the subjects. The success of the subsequent key informant interviews depended on accurate interpretation of the issues.

*Recruitment*

Subjects were recruited through posters centrally displayed in each of four housing complexes. In addition, site staff actively solicited appropriate subjects for the focus groups. Attendance was encouraged through reminder letters distributed to each volunteer 24-hours prior to the meeting.

*Procedure*

All focus groups were held at 9:00 A.M. and typically lasted until 10:30. Two were held in community rooms, one in the library, and one in the arts and crafts room within each complex. Furniture in each of the rooms was moved into an open, group arrangement. A high quality tape recorder and PZM microphone were strategically placed.

Seven to twelve women participated at each site (Table 2). The focus group protocol followed the recommendations of Krueger (1994). (Additional sources of guidance included Greenbaum 1988; Morgan

1988; Shepherd and Achterberg 1992.) The moderator guide is located in Appendix A.

**Table 2: Focus group subjects by site**

| Site | Town | Number in Focus Group | Follow-up Interviews |
|---|---|---|---|
| A | Glastonbury | 12 | 2 |
| B | Norwich | 7 | 1 |
| C | Taftville | 7 | 0 |
| D | Vernon | 9 | 2 |
| Total | | 35 | 5 |

The opening question regarded food likes and dislikes and was followed by successively more focused questions. The sequence is described in Table 3. In general, conversation among the subjects proceeded with minimal guidance from the moderator.

**Table 3: Sequence of questions used to guide focus groups**

| | |
|---|---|
| Opening | First two groups asked about favorite and least liked foods. These questions generated more discussion than desired. For third and fourth group asked what food would you not buy at the grocery store. |
| Introductory | Asked to think of others as well as themselves. What do you consider when deciding what to have for dinner? |
| Transition | Mrs. X mentioned that what you eat should be good for you (or whatever similar phrase was used by Mrs. X). How do you decide what is good for you? |
| Key | Although you know the way you should eat, sometimes you can't. What are some of the reasons you can't eat the things you think you should? |
| Closing | Listed all barriers discussed in response to Key Question. Asked the women to write down on a sheet of paper the top three issues for them personally. Sheets were then collected. |

NOTE: For specifics, please refer to the moderator guide in Appendix A. Method follows recommendations of Krueger 1994.

## Methods

*Text Analysis*

Each session was audiotape recorded and field notes were taken. The tape-based analysis was initiated by listening to each tape at least twice. Verbal passages describing potential barriers to healthful nutrition were transcribed verbatim. The applicable verbal events (content units) ranged from a few sentences to a full page. The transcribers used Word Perfect for text data entry. The files were then pulled into The Ethnograph V4.0 (Seidel, Friese, and Leonard 1995) for further analysis.

The field notes and sketches from listening to the tapes were used to create initial coding categories. Verbal passages were coded, grouped, reduced, recoded, and further reorganized to elucidate the most parsimonious, yet complete, categorization scheme of food and nutrition concerns. The types of situations that create concerns were then condensed into 19 issue statements in the language of the focus group subjects. The results are described more fully in Chapter 3.

## Follow-up Interviews

Individual follow-up interviews with prior subjects are recommended to verify interpretation (Greenbaum 1988). The objectives of the follow-up interviews were to:

- confirm the categorization scheme,
- verify the language of the issue statements, and
- determine if differences in disclosure of nutrition-related problems occurred in the individual situation.

*Recruitment*

One complex did not participate in the follow-up interview process at the request of the Resident Service Coordinator. (She believed that the residents would discern preferential treatment of the selected individuals.) A random sample of 11 subjects was selected from the participants at the remaining three complexes. Letters were mailed to each of the 11 requesting participation in an individual interview. Five individuals agreed to participate.

The five subjects represented all three housing complexes (Table 2). The interviewer subjectively noted that they varied in functional abilities, financial status, education, and social support network properties.

*Procedure*

Each woman was interviewed in her apartment. Field notes were kept but the session was not audio recorded. The nineteen issue statements derived from the focus group discussions were individually typed onto 3x5" cards. The cards were sorted into two piles; one pile consisted of concerns the subject had experienced and the other of concerns she had not experienced. As the cards were being read and sorted a conversational interview was conducted (Weiss 1994). The interviews lasted 45 to 90 minutes.

*Field Note Analyses and Results*

The results of the follow-up interviews indicated that the issue statements were appropriate and on-target for the intended audience. The wording of four of the nineteen statements was altered to improve clarity. In addition, two of the original statements were condensed into one issue. For these women *"all the bother of cooking"* appears tied to cooking *"just for one."* The statement about being *"not sure what I should or shouldn't eat"* was dropped. The interpretation overlapped with other issues in the Food Consumption category. Original and revised statements are shown in Table 4.

**Key Informant Interviews**

The result of the focus groups was a listing of the nutrition concerns of elderly women. The follow-up interviews were used to confirm the concerns and refine issue statements. The issue statements then became the foundation for the open-ended interview with the key informants.

## Table 4: Food and nutrition concerns

| Food Level | Issue Statements (Stressors) |
|---|---|
| Food Acquisition | I don't drive to the grocery store. (Changed from *Getting to the grocery store is a problem*.) <br> These days, food costs too much. <br> Grocery shopping is tiring. (Changed from *Grocery shopping is too tiring*.) <br> They don't sell foods in the small portion sizes I need. |
| (Food Acquisition and Preparation) | Shopping and cooking are difficult because of my disabilities. (Changed from *My health makes it hard to shop and cook*.) |
| Food Preparation | Sometimes I don't feel like going to all the bother of cooking just for myself. (Combined from two statements *Often I don't feel like going to all the bother of cooking*, and *It's hard to cook just for one*.) <br> When I'm sick I don't cook. |
| Food Consumption | I forget to eat meals. <br> I snack too much at night. <br> I eat certain foods to avoid constipation. <br> When I eat away from home, I eat foods that I shouldn't. <br> I have to watch my diet. <br> Deleted: *Sometimes, I'm not sure what I should or shouldn't eat*. <br> Some foods don't agree with me. <br> I am working to lose weight. <br> Foods don't taste as good as they did in the past. <br> When I'm down in the dumps, I don't eat right. (Changed from *When I'm down in the dumps I eat poorly*.) <br> Some foods take too much effort to chew. |

NOTE: Some issue statements were refined after the follow-up interviews and key informant pilot interviews. The original version is shown in italics. Otherwise, the original version was also the final version (normal print).

The primary objective of the key informant interviews was to ascertain the providers and functions of nutrition-related social support. The procedure was revised from the work of Gottlieb (1978) who categorized helping behaviors offered to low-income mothers of young children. The key informant interviews ran through the spring and summer of 1995.

*Recruitment*

The Resident Service Coordinators of the four CHFA housing sites carefully selected the recruits for the key informant interviews. The informants consisted of 16 articulate individuals who met all selection criteria.

*Procedure*

The first four key informant interviews, one from each site, were used as pilots to test the interview guide and the audio taping equipment. The only woman who refused to be audiotaped was the second pilot interview. The pilot interviews resulted in some minor wording changes in the interview schedule (Spradley 1979; Weiss 1994).

The four pilot and 12 subsequent interviews followed the same sequence, which was thoughtfully arranged to encourage participant response. First, mental status was screened to insure data reliability. The open-ended portion of the interview was then conducted, including the problem card sort and the social support interview. The meeting concluded with an assessment of functional status and demographics.

The interviews lasted about two hours, varying from 45 minutes to three and one-half hours. Immediately after the session, field notes were expanded and the interviewer recorded impressions of the informants' affect and any outstanding traits.

Screening

Mental status was ascertained with the Short Portable Mental Status Questionnaire (SPMSQ) (Pfeiffer 1975). Pfeiffer reported acceptable reliability and validity of this instrument. Test-retest reliability at four weeks was 0.82 in 59 individuals age 65 or over. Categorization of mental status by the SPMSQ was in agreement with clinical diagnosis in 81% of 213 subjects.

Further tests of validity and reliability were conducted when the SPMSQ was included in the Older American Resources and Services Program Multidimensional Functional Assessment Questionnaire (OARS OMFAQ) (Fillenbaum 1986). Criterion validity was based on a comparison between SPMSQ results and clinical assessment by geropsychiatrists for 31 subjects. Level of agreement reached 0.60 with

*Methods* 35

Kendall's tau while Spearman's correlation was 0.67. Pearson product moment correlations to assess intra-rater reliability ranged from 0.47 to 0.92 (n=7). Inter-rater reliability was 0.80 (n=11).

Problem card sort

The 17 revised issues statements were typed onto 3x5" cards. The subjects first sorted the cards into two piles representing problems they had experienced and problems they had not experienced. The pile of experienced problems was then divided into another two piles representing major concerns and small issues.

Open-ended social support interview

During the open-ended interview, each of the major concerns was discussed. Appendix B contains the interview guide. Three questions were asked with respect to each concern to explore the types and providers of support.

a. Specifically, who do/did you talk with about this?
b. How has X become involved in helping you deal with the problem or your feelings about it?
c. Is there anything in particular about X as a person or about his/her way of helping you deal with the problem that stands out for you?

Questions b and c are from the work of Gottlieb (1978, 107). Depending on the informant, from three to 17 issues were discussed. The entire open-ended interview was audio recorded using a compact tape recorder. In addition, field notes were maintained.

Functional status

Functional status was defined as the ability to perform typical activities of daily living. Three established instruments were used to assess basic, instrumental, and advanced functional abilities. Table 5 shows the tasks and the references for each instrument.

The scales for both BADL and IADL are included in the OARS OMFAQ (Fillenbaum 1986). Validity and reliability of the combined scales has been assessed. Criterion validity was based on a comparison with clinical assessment by physical therapists for 30 subjects. Level of agreement reached 0.75 with Kendall's tau while Spearman's correlation was 0.82. Pearson product moment correlations to assess intra-rater reliability ranged from 0.78 to 0.92 (n=7). Inter-rater reliability was 0.66 (n=11).

Nagi (1976) does not report reliability statistics for the AADL instrument. The instrument, along with additional items, was administered to a large probability sample of 6493 subjects. The questionnaire results were similar to other national statistics on disability and dependence in living.

**Table 5: Tasks for assessment of functional status**

Basic Activities of Daily Living (BADL) (Katz et al. 1963)
    Eating
    Dressing
    Taking care of appearance, i.e. combing hair
    Walking
    Transferring in and out of bed
    Bathing
    Toileting
Instrumental Activities of Daily Living (IADL) (Lawton and Brody 1969)
    Using telephone
    Using transportation
    Shopping
    Preparing meals
    Performing housework
    Taking medication
    Managing money
Advanced Activities of Daily Living (AADL) (Nagi 1976)
    Walking $1/4$ mile
    Climbing stairs
    Stooping, crouching, kneeling
    Reaching over head
    Using fingers to grasp
    Lifting and carrying 10 pounds

Demographic questionnaire

The demographic questionnaire requested information on ethnicity, age, education, marital status, living situation, health, and rent.

## Text Analyses

The audio tape recordings were transcribed in full and pulled into The Ethnograph v4.0 (Seidel, Friese, and Leonard 1995). Segments of the audiotapes were reviewed multiple times to ensure accuracy in the transcriptions. Additional notes were inserted pertaining to voice tone and observations from the original interview. The original interviewer was the sole analyst of the qualitative data.

The definition of Gottlieb (1978, 107) was used to identify and code all applicable content units.

> The scoring unit consisted of explicit descriptions of the helping behaviors – verbal, action-oriented or material – which were extended and/or the qualities of the helper deemed influential. Statements describing the helper's impact on the respondent, frequently signaled by the stem "X made me feel like . . ." were not acceptable as scoring units.

Furthermore, **the helping behavior had to be linked to an identified nutrition problem**. In addition, the informants occasionally described misguided helping behaviors. These were coded as instances of oversupport and undersupport.

Originally, the categories were coded according to the categorization schema of Gottlieb. However, comparisons within and between coding categories did not appear consistent. Verbal markers were checked; transcripts were examined for missing passages; scoring units were narrowed. Still, interpretation remained ambiguous.

An alternative method of analysis was employed using cut and sort. Previous coding labels were ignored. Passages that appeared to express similar types of helping behaviors were sorted into piles. The groups made conceptual sense. Alternative grouping schemas were arranged. None were as interpretive as the first effort. A few days later, the process was repeated. Again, the first grouping effort of the previous occasion emerged quickly. Case studies of each informant were sketched according to the unfolding schema. The condensed stories appeared to distinctly portray the situation of each individual.

The resultant nutrition-related helping behavior schema is not too dissimilar from the schema identified by Gottlieb (1978). The frequencies and emphases simply differ. Shedding preconceived notions permitted the data to lead (Tesch 1990). The results are discussed in Chapter 4. The findings were used to develop the Nutrition Social Support Questionnaire integral to Phase II.

## PHASE II: STRUCTURED INTERVIEWS

Phase II was initiated to investigate the providers and types of support in a larger sample. Nutrition-related stress and nutrition-related support were simultaneously assessed to determine their direct and interactive relationships with diet quality. Power analysis to determine sample size was not possible as no prior research exists in this area to estimate variance. A sample size of 80 to 100 was presumed sufficient for the multiple regression model.

The recruitment and data collection for the second phase were conducted in conjunction with the Senior Nutrition Awareness Project (SNAP) of the FNP. SNAP was a new nutrition information resource program for low-income elders in Connecticut. The program was being introduced to potential clients in government subsidized housing. While introducing the program, subjects were recruited for a large SNAP research project. The subjects of the social support study consist of a subset of the SNAP research subjects.

The SNAP recruitment and interviewing team included two SNAP staff members and two graduate students. SNAP research staff held training sessions to guarantee that recruitment, interviewing and coding procedures were consistent. Recruitment for Phase II was instituted in December 1995.

### Recruitment

A Housing Directory for Older Adults (CT Department on Aging 1992) and local phone books were used to identify all government subsidized housing sites within a 40-mile radius of Storrs. The original intent was a random sample from resident housing lists. However, public housing officials were not permitted to disclose the names of residents. Thus, an opportunistic sample was recruited via two methods. The first was a mass mailing/survey approach and the second was a simple request for volunteers.

*Methods* 39

*Mass mailing/survey approach*

Letters were hand-delivered twice to 1025 units in 13 housing complexes in six towns. The letters announced the new SNAP program and included a request to complete an enclosed survey. Simultaneously, the program was announced at gatherings, through newsletters, and posters. Appendix C contains an example of the survey.

Overall, 420 surveys were returned for a 41% response rate. Of those, 158 met the gender and age criteria for this study. However of the 158, 56 were not interested in participating in the research project; 36 did not meet additional selection criteria (living situation or functional status), and 5 withdrew part-way through the interview process. Thus, the final sample from the letter/survey method for the social support study was 61 women.[1]

*Request for volunteers*

Because of the arduous nature of the letter/survey method and the low number of actual recruits, supplemental methods of enlisting subjects were sought. The SNAP program was simultaneously recruiting older adults through a volunteer process in additional towns. Resident Service Coordinators encouraged residents to attend SNAP introductory sessions. During the session, SNAP staff asked for volunteers for the research project. Nineteen subjects from 741 units in seven complexes in four towns were recruited for the social support study via the presentation request for volunteers. All 19 completed the interview series.

In addition, letters requesting volunteers for a nutrition study were delivered to 198 units in four small complexes in four towns. Twenty-four women volunteered to participate. However, two appeared mentally incapable. Thus, twenty-two subjects completed interviews for the social support study through the letter request.

The final sample for the social support study consisted of 102 women from 26 complexes in 16 towns.[2] Additional description of the subjects is provided in Chapter 3.

## Procedures

The interview usually took three meetings, following the sequence shown in Table 6. A few women in poor health required shorter interview sessions and subsequently more meetings. Most subjects were interviewed in their apartments. A small number preferred to meet in the community rooms of their buildings.

**Table 6: Structured interview schedule**

Interview 1
    Human subject consent
    Demographic information
    First half of the NCI Food Frequency Questionnaire
    Directions and forms for self-completed questionnaires
Subject self-completed between first and second interview
    Food Behavior Inventory
    NSI DETERMINE Check-list
Interview 2
    Second half of the NCI Food Frequency Questionnaire
    Functional Status
Interview 3
    Nutrition Social Support Questionnaire
    Social Anchorage
    Height and weight

NOTE: Additional information was collected at the first two interviews for the SNAP project. Only information relevant to the social support study is outlined here.

The first two interviews were conducted by either of the two SNAP interviewers or occasionally by one of the graduate students (M.P.). The third interview was conducted by either of the two graduate students. The average time between interviews was 10 days (ranging from 1 to 29 days). High subject retention and compliance were reinforced with reminder telephone calls the day before each interview.

*Data Collected*

The questionnaires used in Phase II are described below.

## National Cancer Institute (NCI) Food Frequency Questionnaire

Since both sources of stress in this study are chronic situations, the measure of diet quality needed to reflect long-term intake. Thus, the National Cancer Institute Food Frequency Questionnaire (Block et al. 1986) was selected to assess habitual intake over the past year. Reliability and validity of this instrument have been evaluated in numerous studies (Block et al. 1990; Block and Hartman 1989; Cummings et al. 1987; and Mares-Perlman et al. 1993). Test-retest reliability for nutrient values averages 0.70. Validity is generally evaluated from comparisons with results from food records. Correlations between nutrient values from the two methods generally range from 0.5 to 0.6. The strength of the correlation varies by nutrient as well as the number of food record days.

Prior to implementing Phase II, the food frequency questionnaire was revised for use with older adults. For instance, specific queries regarding cranberry juice, prunes, and beets were added, while other specific food items were deleted, such as pumpkin pie.[3] A section on low-fat food usage was expanded from the original version, as recommended by Patterson, Haines, and Popkin (1996).

The modified version asked about the frequency of eating 93 items. Subjects indicated the portion sizes as small, medium, or large. The respondents were also asked to report consumption of any additional foods consumed more than once per month. Furthermore, information was collected regarding usual food practices, such as frequency of eating away from home and type of cooking fat.

## Food Behavior Inventory

The Food Behavior Inventory (FBI) (Fey-Yensan 1995) is a list of 98 specific food behaviors, such as *"I eat a snack before supper."* Respondents rank the frequency with which they perform each behavior (Appendix D). Factor analysis revealed that the instrument examines eight distinct factors: interest in cooking, eating enjoyment, food-related dependence, healthy food practices, meal routine, use of canned/frozen foods, social eating, and overeating. Internal reliability estimates for seven of the eight factors exceeded 0.70. External validity was examined in a group of 60 independently living elderly women. Food patterns and BMI paralleled the results of the FBI.

NSI DETERMINE Check-list

The NSI DETERMINE checklist (Lipschitz and White 1991) was developed to increase awareness of the importance of good nutrition for elderly persons. The self-administered questionnaire assesses 10 warning signs of poor nutritional status. The NSI has established a weighted scoring method to calculate a total risk score.

Demographic information and Functional status

The demographic information and functional status were assessed exactly as in the key informant interviews, previously discussed.

Nutrition Social Support Questionnaire

The Nutrition Social Support Questionnaire was developed from the results of Phase I. The questionnaire inquires about the general support network, including both received and reciprocal support, and the nutrition-specific support network. The main focus of the questionnaire is on the providers and functions of social support in response to food acquisition, food preparation, and food consumption needs (Appendix E).

Social Anchorage

Social anchorage is the degree to which an individual feels embedded in her community. Social anchorage was assessed using the eight-item scale developed by Hanson and Ostergren (1987). These researchers assessed test-retest reliability of their instrument after three weeks in 30 men. Agreement for the individual questionnaire items ranged from 79% to 97%. Construct validity was inferred from associations with marital status and nervous problems in 500 men.

Height and weight

Height was measured against a wall using a standard, nonstretchable tape measure. In the only case in which standing height was not possible, height was calculated from knee height (Haboubi, Hudson, and Pathy 1990). Weight was measured using a Health-O-Meter

## Methods

Ultrapro Professional Dial Scale. Height and weight were each measured three times or until results were consistent.

*Outcome Measures*

The descriptive and analytic outcome variables are listed in Table 7. Operational definitions of the measures of diet quality, nutrition stress, and nutrition-related social support follow. Further specifics regarding the calibrations of each measure are included in the chapters of results. Diet quality was derived from analysis of the NCI food frequency questionnaire (Block et al. 1986). The data for the social support and diet variables were collected in the nutrition social support questionnaire.

**Table 7: Descriptive and analytic outcome variables**

|  | Descriptive | Analytic Dependent | Analytic Independent |
|---|---|---|---|
| 1 Diet Quality |  |  |  |
| a) Macro and micro nutrient intakes | X |  |  |
| b) Summary measures |  |  |  |
| i) Mean Adequacy Ratio (MAR) |  | X |  |
| ii) Diet Quality Index (DQI) |  | X |  |
| 2 Nutrition Stressors |  |  |  |
| a) Modified diet | X |  |  |
| b) Functional status | X |  | X |
| 3 Nutrition-related Social Support |  |  |  |
| a) Relationships of helpers | X |  |  |
| b) Types of support | X |  |  |
| c) Summary measures |  |  |  |
| i) Total number helpers |  |  | X |
| ii) Total number types |  |  | X |
| iii) Helpers + types |  |  | X |
| d) Satisfaction with support | X |  | X |

Diet Quality

*Macro and micro nutrient intakes:* Vitamins A, C, and E, thiamin, riboflavin, niacin, B6, and folacin, and the minerals calcium, zinc, sodium, phosphorus, magnesium, and iron were analyzed. In addition, total calories, fat, saturated fat, cholesterol, alcohol, protein, carbohydrate, and the percent contribution of each to the total diet were calculated. Dietary fiber intake was also assessed (Smucker et al. 1989).

*Mean Adequacy Ratio (MAR):* MAR is a summary measure of nutrient intake. MAR is the average of the ratio of 11 nutrients relative to the Recommended Dietary Allowance of each (Guthrie and Scheer 1981).

*Diet Quality Index (DQI):* The DQI is a summary diet score based on the 1989 National Academy of Sciences recommendations in *Diet and Health*. The diet is rated on eight dimensions, including percent fat, percent saturated fat, cholesterol, fruit & vegetable intake, complex carbohydrate servings, protein, sodium, and calcium. Scores are totaled and may range from 0 to 16 (Patterson, Haines, and Popkin 1994).

Nutrition Stressors

*Modified diet:* Modified diet was a dichotomous variable. Subjects were considered to follow a modified diet if they reported any type of physician or self-prescribed food regime.

*Functional status:* Four tiers of functional status were identified: 1) individuals with no impairments, 2) individuals with at least one AADL (Nagi 1976) impairment, but no IADL (Lawton and Brody 1969) or BADL (Katz et al. 1963) impairments, 3) individuals with at least one IADL impairment, but no BADL disabilities, and 4) individuals who could not perform at least one BADL without help.

Nutrition-related Social Support

*Relationships of helpers (formal and informal):* Support providers were categorized by relationship, such as daughter, son, or social worker. Furthermore, categories were dichotomized as formal or informal.

*Types of support:* The types of nutrition-related social support were identified during the key informant interviews. Instrumental support is offered in response to food acquisition needs, and includes activities such as transportation to the grocery store or picking up small items, like milk or bread. Informational and emotional support are offered in response to modified diet needs. Helping behaviors such as diet education, encouragement, and reassurance are included.

*Total number helpers:* The total number of persons providing support for each stressor.

*Total number types:* The total number of types being provided for each stressor.

*Helpers + types:* The total number of types across all helpers for each stressor.

*Satisfaction with support:* Subjects reported their current level of satisfaction with nutrition-related support in response to each stressor.

## Data Analyses

Food frequency data were entered and verified using DIETSYS and nutrient analyses were run with DIETANAL of the NCI Food Frequency package (Smucker et al. 1989). The nutrient values of 10 additional foods that the women reported eating, but were not in the NCI database, were added to the data set. Demographic and social support data were entered and verified using Epi Info V6.0 (Dean et al. 1994). Data were uploaded to the University of Connecticut IBM 9021 mainframe computer system. Outlier and influence analyses were run using BMDP (BMDP 1990). Measures of association were run using SAS V6.09 (SAS 1996).

Frequencies and cross-tabulations were used to describe the findings. Correlations were utilized to evaluate the association between measures of social support and functional status. The relationship between functional status and diet quality was examined using bivariate regression. Social support and an interaction term were then added to the equations to investigate the multivariate relationships. Results were considered statistically significant at $p < 0.05$.

## NOTES

1. The most frequent reasons for not participating were "too ill", "too busy", or "not interested." Recruitment survey results were available for 97 nonrespondents who matched the study sample on gender and age. Chi-square analyses indicated no differences between the two groups on self-rated health, modified diets, or diet quality.

2. A comparison between the 61 letter/survey recruited and the 41 volunteer recruited was completed. No difference between the groups exists on self-rated health, functional status, education, BMI, age, years lived alone, or years lived in present complex. The volunteer group does pay significantly higher rents, indicating higher incomes. Although all subjects are low-income

and live in government subsidized housing, the complexes where volunteers were recruited coincidentally appear to be located in higher SES areas than the complexes involved in the letter/survey approach.

3. The NCI food frequency questionnaire was carefully developed to reliably assess the nutrient content of the typical diet. Block et al. (1986) spent considerable effort in selecting which foods to include on the questionnaire. The resultant list contains those items able to account for at least 90% of the total intake of 17 vitamins and minerals, according to the results of NHANES II.

However, the typical diet of any subgroup of the population is likely to be unique in some respects. For example, the high consumption of cranberry juice by the subjects in this study warranted its inclusion on the food list. Simultaneously, the list needed to remain within a reasonable length to avoid over-reporting. Thus some foods had to be deleted. Changes to the list for the purposes of this study were based on findings during the pilot phase, food records maintained by elderly women in the chemosensory study conducted by Duffy (1993) at the University of Connecticut, and reports of food patterns of the elderly in the nutrition literature.

CHAPTER 3
# Description of the Subjects

The subject recruitment and selection criteria for this study were carefully designed to maximize interpretation of the results. Certain characteristics of the participants were held within thoughtfully identified ranges. For instance, all the subjects are women, age 75 to 95 years, living in government subsidized housing. These restrictions permit control of factors that might obscure the ability to discern relationships between the primary variables of interest.

In contrast, a normal distribution on other characteristics of the respondents was desirable. Specifically, functional status, physical health, and dietary patterns of the subjects needed to correspond to a larger population of elderly women. A similar match between sample and population permits greater generalizability, and thus applicability.

Below, the demographic characteristics and physical health indices of this sample are described. Simultaneously, national data and results from similar studies are compared to subject characteristics.

## DEMOGRAPHICS

The oldest age groups are the fastest growing segment of the United States population (Siegel 1993). The 1990 census data indicated that 5.8% of the Connecticut population was 75 years or over (U.S. Bureau of the Census 1992). This proportion is expected to climb until the year 2040, at which time forecasters anticipate that the age group will stabilize at 12% of the population (Siegel 1993). In Connecticut in 1990, more than two out of every three persons over 75 years were female (U.S. Bureau of the Census 1992). While 91% of the women age 75 to 84 years were living independently, the proportion dropped to only 67% of those 85 years or over.

Both food patterns and characteristics of social support vary with gender. To control this influence, only females were recruited for this study. As a further control, currently married or recently widowed females were excluded. Table 8 shows the marital status of the subjects in the three interviewing activities. The majority were widowed. Because of the inclusion criteria, the proportion of widowed and divorced subjects was higher than that in the general U.S. population for women over 75 years (Saluter 1996).

**Table 8: Marital status**

|  | Phase I | | Phase II |
|---|---|---|---|
|  | Focus Groups (n=35) | Key Informants (n=12) | Comprehensive (n=102) |
| Single (always) | 0 | 0 | 6 |
| Widowed | 32 | 12 | 82 |
| Divorced | 1 | 0 | 14 |
| Not answered | 2 | 0 | 0 |

Table 9 shows ethnicity, education and town of residence of subjects. Over $3/4$ of the subjects report five to twelve years of education. A smaller proportion of women received higher education than in the general Connecticut population. U.S. census data indicate that 21% of Connecticut residents over 75 years have received from 1 year of college to advanced degrees (U.S. Bureau of the Census 1993). Only 10% of these subjects progressed beyond high school.

Respondents were recruited from small to moderate size towns within a one-hour driving distance from the University of Connecticut. The response rate was similar among housing complexes involved in similar recruitment strategies. Thus, the larger towns are represented in the same proportion as the smaller towns. The greater absolute number of respondents from the larger towns is merely a reflection of the population distribution.

## Table 9: Ethnicity, education, and town of residence

|  | Phase I | | Phase II |
|---|---|---|---|
|  | Focus Groups (n=35) | Key Informants (n=12) | Comprehensive (n=102) |
| **Ethnicity** | | | |
| White | 33 | 11 | 100 |
| African-American | 1 | 1 | 2 |
| Latino-American | 1 | 0 | 0 |
| **Education** | | | |
| 0–4 years | 1 | 1 | 1 |
| 5–8 years | 8 | 5 | 30 |
| some High School | 8 | 2 | 18 |
| H.S. graduate | 7 | 3 | 29 |
| Business/Trade | 0 | 0 | 14 |
| 1–3 years College | 8 | 1 | 5 |
| College graduate | 2 | 0 | 3 |
| Graduate degree | 0 | 0 | 2 |
| Not answered | 1 | 0 | 0 |
| **Town of Residence** | | | |
| (# complexes) | | | |
| Bloomfield (2) | 0 | 0 | 10 |
| Colchester (2) | 0 | 0 | 2 |
| Coventry (1) | 0 | 0 | 8 |
| Ellington (1) | 0 | 0 | 5 |
| Glastonbury (2) | 12 | 3 | 3 |
| Groton (1) | 0 | 0 | 4 |
| Manchester (4) | 0 | 0 | 25 |
| New London (1) | 0 | 0 | 2 |
| Norwich (3) | 7 | 3 | 3 |
| Rockville (1) | 9 | 3 | 0 |
| Stafford Springs (1) | 0 | 0 | 5 |
| Taftville (1) | 7 | 3 | 0 |
| Talcotville (1) | 0 | 0 | 12 |
| Tolland (1) | 0 | 0 | 4 |
| Willimantic (3) | 0 | 0 | 18 |
| Woodstock (1) | 0 | 0 | 1 |

A further description of the subjects is shown in Table 10. The overall mean age is 81 years, ranging from 75 to 95 years. The minimum number of years living alone is five, but most of the subjects have lived alone at least two decades. The minimum number of years living at the present apartment is two, with a mean of approximately ten years.

**Table 10: Age and living situation**

|  | Phase I | | Phase II |
|---|---|---|---|
|  | Focus Groups (n=32) mean±SD | Key Informants (n=12) mean±SD | Comprehensive (n=102) mean±SD |
| Age | 79.2±3.8 | 79.2±2.4 | 82.2±4.7 |
| (Range) | (75–88) | (75–82) | (75–95) |
| Years alone | 20.5±12.3 | 16.4±9.6 | 22.4±11.4 |
| Years at complex | 9.5±4.9 | 9.1±3.9 | 11.9±6.2 |

All of the subjects live in government subsidized housing. In these units, rent is generally about 33% of total income.[1] Table 11 shows the rent categories of the respondents. The estimated income of almost 75% of the subjects falls below the 1996 poverty level (U.S. DHHS 1996).

**Table 11: Monthly rent**

|  | Phase I | | Phase II |
|---|---|---|---|
| Rent ($) | Focus Groups (n=35) | Key Informants (n=12) | Comprehensive (n=102) |
| ≤ 99 | 0 | 0 | 17 |
| 100–199 | 16 | 7 | 48 |
| 200–299 | 10 | 4 | 18 |
| 300–399 | 5 | 1 | 12 |
| 400 + | 3 | 0 | 4 |
| Not answered | 1 | 0 | 3 |

Elderly females are one of the poorest subgroups of the U.S. population (U.S. Bureau of the Census 1996). In 1990, 18% of Connecticut residents 75 years or older had incomes below the poverty level; slightly over 50% were below 150% of the poverty level (U.S. Bureau of the Census 1993). As these statistics include both sexes, the poverty rate for females alone would be even higher. Judging by U.S. population figures, approximately $1/4$ of all single living elderly women have incomes below poverty level (Hansson and Carpenter 1994; Iams and Sandell 1995).

Residence in government subsidized housing has implications beyond economic insufficiency. The effects on social support are also of concern for the purposes of this study. Initially, policy-makers and researchers speculated that the relative age homogeneity of the living situation would encourage social interaction between residents. In agreement, when residents are looked at en mass, social contact with neighbors is positively related to age density of the environment (Hinrichsen 1985; Poulin 1984). However, the preponderance of social interaction is conducted between the healthy residents of the complex. Frail elders receive substantially less support from neighbors than their healthy counterparts (Kaye and Monk 1991; Sheehan 1986).

Over time, changes have occurred in the social environment of public housing complexes for the elderly (Golant 1992; Karasik 1989). Residents have "aged in place," resulting in greater numbers of frail occupants. Disabled young adults have also been integrated into the complexes. Concern over crime, either adjacent to or within the complex, has risen. These changes may increase social isolation among residents.

## HEALTH

Table 12 shows the self-reported health and illnesses of the subjects. About 60% of the women reported "good" health and about 30% reported "fair" health. This distribution of responses is similar to the results of other, larger surveys (Siegel 1993). Arthritis is generally the most frequently cited condition by women in this age group (U.S. Bureau of the Census 1996). Hypertension is the second most common, with heart conditions following closely.

These chronic conditions become more common with increasing age. However, while the medical diagnoses may be similar, the impact of the illness differs depending on the individual (Dwyer 1995). Stage of illness, economic resources, and psychological and physiological adaptations influence the ability to carry out daily tasks. Thus, the impact of the condition is often assessed in terms of the impact on functional status, or the ability to carry out self-care and home management activities.

### Table 12: Self-reported health and self-reported illness

|  | Phase I | | Phase II |
|---|---|---|---|
|  | Focus Groups (n=35) | Key Informants (n=12) | Comprehensive (n=102) |
| **Health** | | | |
| Excellent | 1 | 2 | 7 |
| Good | 20 | 1 | 60 |
| Fair | 13 | 6 | 27 |
| Poor | 0 | 3 | 8 |
| Not answered | 1 | 0 | 0 |
| **Illnesses** [a] | | | |
| Arthritis | 11 | 3 | 57 |
| Diabetes | 5 | 4 | 4 |
| Heart disease | 11 | 4 | 40 |
| Hypertension | 14 | 6 | 48 |
| G.I. disorders | 2 | 3 | 29 |
| Osteoporosis | 1 | 2 | 6 |
| Vision difficulties | 0 | 4 | 23 |

[a] Over 80% of the subjects reported more than one illness. Therefore, numbers in columns add to more than 100%.

## Functional Status

The capabilities of elderly individuals fluctuate for better and worse over time, due to illnesses, rehabilitative efforts, new adaptations, occurrence of additional life stressors, remissions, or other influences (Crimmins and Saito 1993; Smith et al. 1990). However, for the elderly as a group, functional status shows a gradual decline with advancing age (Kovar, Hendershot, and Mathis 1989). Lower functional status is associated with increased risk of mortality even when age is statistically controlled (Reuben et al. 1992).

Functional status for the key informants and the comprehensive interview groups was assessed using three scales – the Basic Activities of Daily Living (BADL) (Katz et al. 1963), the Instrumental Activities of Daily Living (IADL) (Lawton and Brody 1969), and the Advanced Activities of Daily Living (AADL) (Nagi 1976). The BADLs are tasks that are essential for daily life, such as the ability to eat and to get out of bed. The IADLs are slightly higher level skills, such as using the

*Description of the Subjects* 53

telephone, taking medications, and preparing meals. The AADLs are activities that are helpful, but not essential for daily living, such as walking up 10 stair steps without resting, and reaching up overhead.

Subjects were categorized into one of four tiers of functional ability. The tiers, from highest functioning to most disabled, are as follows (Fitti and Kovar 1992):

- NO DISABILITIES: no reported difficulties at any level;
- AADL DISABILITIES: reported difficulty with at least one advanced activity of daily living, such as carrying something as heavy as 10 pounds or walking $1/4$ mile, but no reported difficulties with IADLs or BADLs;
- IADL DISABILITIES: reported difficulty with at least one instrumental activity of daily living, such as preparing meals, managing money or shopping, but no reported difficulty with BADLs;
- BADL DISABILITIES: reported difficulty with at least one basic activity of daily living, such as bathing, dressing or transferring out of bed.

The hierarchical nature of these abilities has been explored with data from the Longitudinal Study on Aging (Crimmins and Saito 1993). Using the same categories, Harris et al. (1989) found that higher disability levels were associated with increased morbidity and mortality over a two-year period. Table 13 shows the functional status categories of the subjects in this study.

**Table 13: Functional status**

|  | Phase I<br>Key Informants<br>(n=12) | Phase II<br>Comprehensive<br>(n=102) |
|---|---|---|
| No disabilities | 1 | 13 |
| AADL disabilities | 3 | 27 |
| IADL disabilities | 2 | 29 |
| BADL disabilities | 6 | 33 |

The most common difficulties for the respondents are stooping, crouching, or kneeling (69%) and lifting or carrying something as heavy as 10 pounds (63%). Over fifty percent report difficulty walking

2 to 3 blocks, walking up 10 stair steps, and doing heavy housework, such as washing curtains and windows. All these activities, except for the housework, are included on the advanced scale.

The National Health Interview Survey, Supplement on Aging (LSOA), conducted in 1984, measured these same three levels of functional abilities in a national probability sample of older adults. The proportion of women in this study reporting difficulty with each of the AADLs is similar to the proportion in the national probability sample (Kovar, Weeks, and Forbes 1995). Some of the questions regarding the IADLs and BADLs differ between this study and the LSOA. For the questions that are comparable, the proportions of women needing help with the activities is again similar (Fulton et al. 1989). The distribution of disabilities also corresponds to the 1992 census results (U.S. Bureau of the Census 1996). Table 14 shows a comparison between samples.

**Table 14: Activities of daily living (ADLs)—comparison with national data**

| Activities of Daily Living | Nationally Representative Samples | | This study (%) |
|---|---|---|---|
| | 1985 NHIS [a] (%) | 1991 Census [b] (%) | |
| Advanced ADLs | | | |
| Walk a quarter mile | 67 | | 50 |
| Walk up 10 steps – no rest | 53 | | 50 |
| Stoop, crouch, or kneel | 72 | | 69 |
| Reach up over head | 28 | | 33 |
| Use fingers to grasp | 16 | | 28 |
| Lift and carry 10 pounds | 41 | | 63 |

*Description of the Subjects* 55

**Table 14 continued**

| Activities of Daily Living | Nationally Representative Samples | | This study (%) |
|---|---|---|---|
| | 1985 NHIS [a] (%) | 1991 Census [b] (%) | |
| Instrumental ADLs | | | |
| Use telephone | | 8 | 5 |
| Get outside | | 26 | 26 |
| Shop | 16 | | 30 |
| Perform heavy housework | 66 | | 50 |
| Prepare meals | 8 | 14 | 10 |
| Handle own money | 7 | 12 | 14 |
| Basic ADLs | | | |
| Eat | 2 | 3 | 0 |
| Dress | 7 | 8 | 1 |
| Walk | | 20 | 11 |
| Transfer | 5 | 13 | 4 |
| Bathe | 12 | 13 | 28 |

[a] The NHIS employed complex weighting procedures to accurately project the results from their sample to U.S. citizens as a whole. The national probability sample included 2650 women age 75+. References for this information include Fulton et al. 1989 and Kovar, Weeks, and Forbes 1995.

[b] Estimates were calculated by the Census Bureau from unpublished statistics of wave 3 of the 1991 Survey of Income and Program Participation (U.S. Bureau of the Census 1996). Again, complex regression methods were used with the nationally representative, weighted sample.

In summary, the range and types of physical capabilities reported by the recruits for this study appear to be representative of the U.S. population of women age 75 or over.

## Body Mass Index (BMI)

During Phase II, the interviewer measured the heights and weights of the subjects. Standing height was assessed against a wall using a standard, nonstretchable tape measure. (In one case, knee height was measured and standing height was calculated [Haboubi, Hudson, and

Pathy 1990]). Weight was measured using a Health-O-Meter Ultrapro Professional dial scale. Table 15 shows the results of these measures.

**Table 15: Height, weight, and Body Mass Index**

|  | Phase II Comprehensive (n=100)[a] | | |
|---|---|---|---|
|  | Mean | SD | Range |
| Height (inches) | 60.9 | 2.0 | (57–66) |
| Weight (pounds) | 149.8 | 31.2 | (76–250) |
| BMI (kg/m$^2$) | 28.4 | 5.7 | (14.5–48.1) |

[a] Missing data from 2 of the total 102 subjects.

Quetelet's index was used to calculate Body Mass Index (BMI) (Abernathy 1991). Currently, BMI reference criteria for older persons are being debated. However, the National Research Council's Committee on Diet and Health suggested that a BMI greater than 29 be used to indicate obesity and associated health risk (Abernathy 1991; White 1991). A BMI less than 24 would indicate an undesirably low weight for height. The recommendation of 24 to 29 is based on age-specific prevalence rates and mortality data and is higher than the recommended range for younger adults. Using the criteria for older adults 19% of the subjects are underweight and 39% are obese (Figure 2).

The average BMI of the subjects in this study is higher than the national mean of 25.9 (+/- 4.5 SD) reported for women 65–85 years in the NHANES I follow-up study (1982–84) (Galanos et al. 1994). The BMI of participants in the NHANES III ( Phase I: 1988–91) averaged 26.7 and 24.6 for women age 70 to 79 and 80+, respectively (Kuczmarski 1998). Other researchers have also reported a lower average BMI in their samples in comparison to the mean of this group (Table 16).

**Figure 2: Distribution on Body Mass Index. (Data missing on two subjects [n=100])**

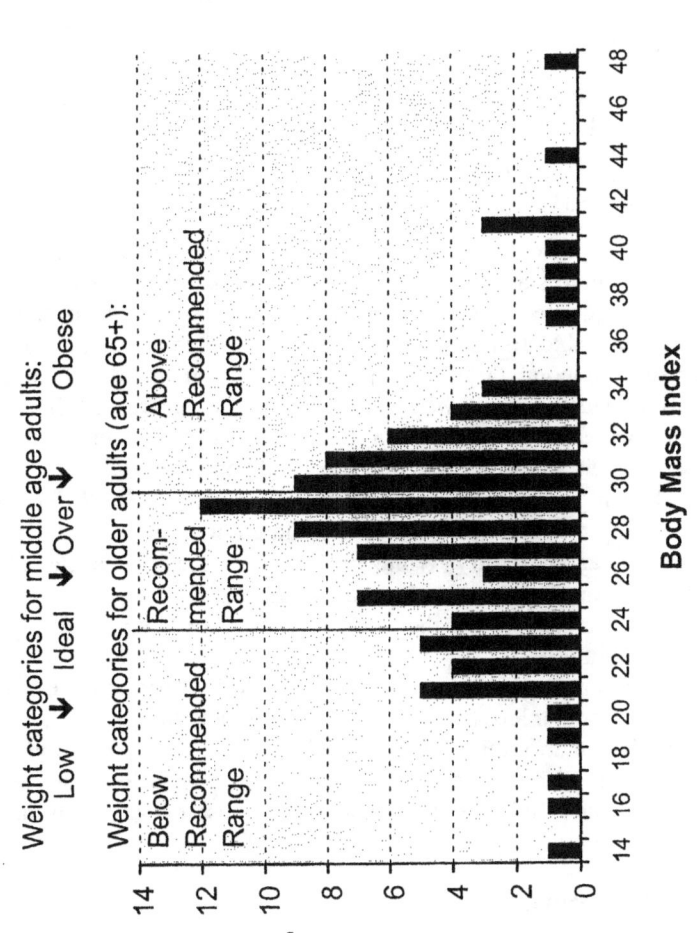

**Table 16: Body Mass Index values reported in the literature**

|  | Sample | BMI ± SD | Location |
|---|---|---|---|
| This study | 100 F 75–95 years | 28.4 ± 5.7 | Connecticut |
| Kubena–1991 | 93 F ≥75 years | 25.1 ± 0.5 (SEM)[a] | Texas |
| Minten–1991 | 250 F 65–79 years | 27.1 ± 4.3 | Netherlands |
| Mowe–1994 | 52 F ≥70 years | 25.4 ± 3.9 | Norway |
| Payette–1995 | 103 F ≥ 60 years | 27.7 ± 7.6 | Canada |
| Roubenoff–1995 | 176 F 70–79 years | 27.9 ± 5.5 | Framingham |
| Roubenoff–1995 | 87 F 80+ years | 27.3 ± 4.5 | Framingham |
| Sem–1988 | 201 F ≥75 years | 22.9 ± NA | Norway |
| Zipp–1992 | 100 F ≥ 65 years | 23.5 ± NA | Kansas |

[a] SEM reported by the authors rather than SD.

The high incidence of obesity in this sample is likely related to the low economic status of the group. Low-income is associated with a higher incidence of obesity in women (Ham 1991). None of the other studies in Table 16 included exclusively low-income samples. In fact, Zipp and Holcomb (1992, 15) were careful to point out that their results profile "*healthy, physically active, highly educated, and financially secure women.*" In comparison, the subjects of this study were more disabled, fairly inactive, less educated, and poorer.

The high incidence of obesity is a concern. A BMI over 30 complicates healthcare and is associated with increased risks of morbidity and mortality (White 1991). Severe obesity is affiliated with hypertension, non-insulin dependent diabetes mellitus, osteoarthritis, and specific cancers. Furthermore, massive obesity appears to predict earlier mortality.

Low body weight is also undesirable. A BMI below 24, especially when accompanied by recent, unintentional weight loss, is also predictive of mortality (Fischer and Johnson 1990). A low BMI is associated with increased probability of hospitalization (Mowe, Bohmer, and Kindt 1994) and with longer hospital stays (Fischer and Johnson 1990).

## NUTRITIONAL RISK

The Nutrition Screening Initiative (NSI) is a collaborative project of the American Dietetic Association, the American Academy of Family

*Description of the Subjects*

Physicians, and the National Council on the Aging. The overall goal of this national effort is to promote nutrition screening and optimal nutrition care for all elderly persons in the United States (White 1991). To meet their goal, the NSI has documented nutritional risk factors, established screening tools, and recommended appropriate nutrition strategies.

The DETERMINE checklist was developed as a first-line screening and awareness tool. The simple questionnaire assesses 10 warning signs for poor nutritional status. The tool was designed to be self-administered by older adults or their caregivers (Lipschitz 1991).

The warning signs include some of the demographic indices that have been discussed previously in this chapter, including social isolation, weight loss, economic hardship, poor health, and physical disability. In addition, the checklist inquires about dietary indicators, such as limited fruit and vegetable consumption and skipping meals.

The NSI established a weighted scoring method for the DETERMINE checklist to calculate a total risk score. The percent of women in each risk category is shown in Table 17. The results from a large Wisconsin study are shown for comparison (Vailas et al. 1997). The risk distribution of the women in this study logically falls between the Wisconsin congregate and home delivered meal participants.

**Table 17: Nutrition Screening Initiative (NSI) DETERMINE checklist scores—in comparison to the findings of Vailas et al. (1997)**

|  | Subject Characteristics | Nutritional Risk (%) | | |
| --- | --- | --- | --- | --- |
|  |  | Low | Mod. | High |
| This study | 102 F, age 75–95 | 28 | 36 | 35 |
| Vailas et al. 1997 | Congregate meal participants, 10,343 F, age 60+ | 48 | 31 | 21 |
|  | Home delivered meal participants, 3,580 F, age 60+ | 15 | 37 | 48 |

Sahyoun et al. (1997) caution that the DETERMINE checklist was developed as a promotional and educational tool. These researchers documented that three of the checklist items are strongly indicative of subsequent mortality, while the overall score is only mildly indicative of mortality. The other seven items are not related to mortality. The high mortality indicators include eating alone, taking multiple medications, and difficulty with shopping and cooking.

Almost 90% of the women in this study report that they eat alone most of the time and 68% take three or more medications daily. In other words, the number of women at moderate and high risk of malnutrition may underestimate the gravity of the situation.

## SOCIAL ANCHORAGE

Social anchorage is defined by Hanson, Mattisson, and Steen (1987, 55) as the *"degree of the individual's sense of belonging to and being part of his community."* Social anchorage was assessed as an indicator of social isolation. The results are shown in Figure 3. Total scores spanned the range of the scale from 0 (absolutely no feeling of belonging) to 8 (firmly embedded in the community).

The distribution of scores was very similar to that reported by Hanson and Ostergren (1987) in their representative sample of 500 68–year-old men in Malmo, Sweden. However, Hanson and Ostergren did note that nonsubjects in their study were more likely to live alone, report poorer health, and be registered with the Temperance Board. Possible under-representation of socially isolated individuals should also be considered when examining the results of this research.

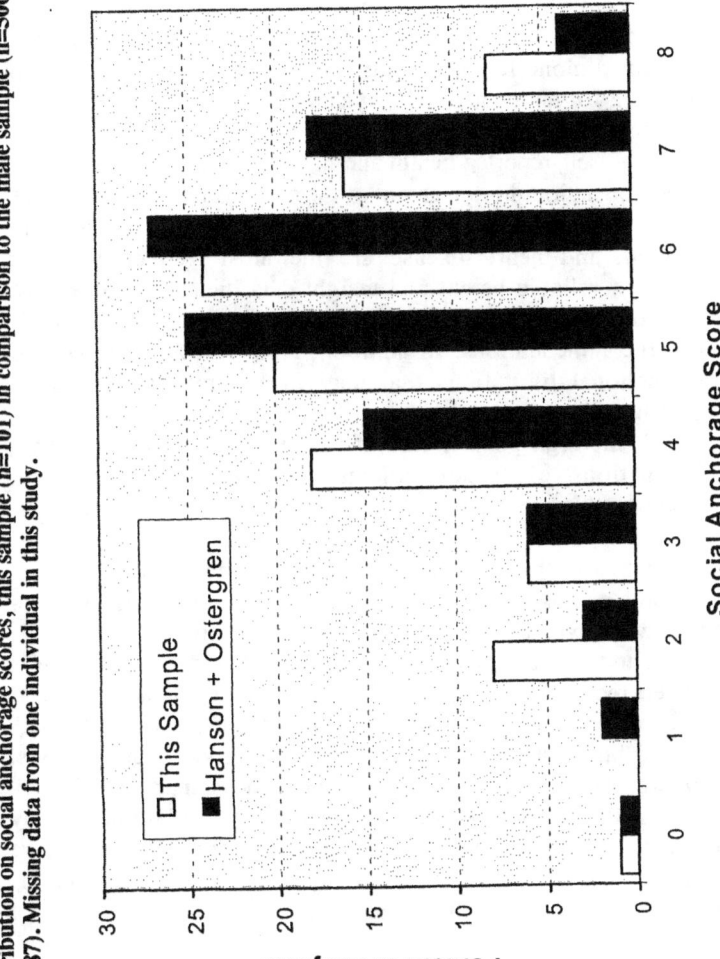

Figure 3: Distribution on social anchorage scores, this sample (n=101) in comparison to the male sample (n=500) of Hanson and Ostergren (1987). Missing data from one individual in this study.

## CONCLUSION

In the next 40 years, the proportion of older adults is expected to double. Currently, two out of every three persons over 75 years of age are female. Most live independently, although as age increases, so does the chance of living in a group situation.

Because of the selection criteria for this study, the subjects are all women, 75 to 95 years old, living in fairly stable situations. As a group, they have lived alone for an average of 20 years and have lived in senior housing for an average of 10 years. Almost $3/4$ have estimated incomes below the poverty line.

In general, self-reported health and illnesses appear similar to that of the U.S. population. Forty percent of the subjects rate their health as fair to poor. Over 95% report one illness or more; arthritis, hypertension, and heart disease are the most frequently cited. Assessment of reliable height and weight data indicates that almost two-thirds of the subjects are at nutritional risk according to BMI reference recommendations. In addition, almost 90% have mild to severe functional limitations that may further negatively impact nutritional status.

Overall, the high poverty rate, the poor health, and the solitary living situations of these subjects presents a grim picture. Unfortunately, this picture is real for a large number of Connecticut residents, as supported by U.S. population statistics.

The women in this sample exemplify the "graying of America." This on-going demographic shift is characterized by growing numbers of elders with extended life expectancy, reduced economic self-sufficiency, and increased chronic and degenerative diseases (Kinsella 1995). Their reduced functional abilities necessitate reliance on social support. However, simultaneous with the upswing in numbers of elders is a reduced birth rate. Of concern are declining kin support ratios. Furthermore, kin are often living greater distances apart, which may impede the ability to provide necessary help. To exacerbate an already worrisome situation, funding is becoming scarce for public health care programs. When informal support is not adequate, formal support becomes a necessary supplement or substitute.

Many of the women in this study look to others for help. Through the interview process they shared their situations and their solutions. By learning more about existing patterns, the ability to identify vulnerable elders in the future is improved. The remainder of this report examines the types and providers of nutrition-related social support as perceived by the older adult respondents in this study. Furthermore, the relationship between social support and dietary quality in this sample is reported.

The generalizability of the results is limited to women over 75 years of age living alone in government subsidized housing. The sample appears representative on the distribution of health, functional status, and nutritional risk in this population. However, socially isolated individuals may be underrepresented. Thus, the frequencies of support are likely to be overestimates for the total population.

## NOTE

1. Government subsidized housing for the elderly refers to a heterogeneous collection of complexes subsidized by one or more federal, state, or local programs. Residents must meet certain age and income eligibility guidelines. However, the complexes vary in a number of ways dependent on the funding source and the administration (Golant 1992).

Construction and upkeep differ, including the percent efficiency units, landscaping, handicap accessibility, and security. Some complexes have one or more community rooms; such as activity rooms, libraries, and dining areas; others have none. Some have services, such as Resident Service Coordinators, buses, congregate meals, and resident programs; others have none. Furthermore, the percent of nonelderly, disabled residents is variable.

Funding, location, and service availability also influence rents (Golant 1992). The proportion of rent from income reported here was calculated from the full SNAP study (n=247) which collected additional data regarding economic resources.

CHAPTER 4
# Nutrition-Related Concerns and Proffered Help

The first objective of this study was to develop a classification scheme of nutrition-related helping behaviors. Prior to examining helping behaviors, the problems perceived by elderly women needed to be ascertained.

The following discussion describes the results of focus group meetings and key informant interviews. The primary goal of the focus groups was to determine typical barriers to good nutrition. Although the language and terminology may differ, the worries of these women are similar to concerns expressed by health care professionals.

After identification of problems, the key informant interviews were conducted to learn about the types and providers of nutrition help. The open-ended interviews resulted in rich descriptions of each subject's unique situation. Content analyses revealed common modes of help specific to each type of problem. From the analysis an overall schema of nutrition-related helping behaviors was developed. The description of helping behaviors and the categorization schema are presented following discussion of perceived problems.

## THE ISSUES

Help is offered in response to a need. Early pilot work for this study demonstrated that elderly women must first perceive that they have the need before they are able to recognize proffered support. For instance, one severely underweight woman did not agree with her physician's recommendation for weight gain. Accordingly, she did not perceive the high calorie recipes he gave her as helpful, nor did she interpret her daughter's frequent delivery of donuts as supportive. Actually, she viewed the donuts as wasted spending, which irritated her.

While the academic literature refers to multiple nutrition problems of elderly persons, the actual perceptions of older adults could differ. Thus, focus groups were held to uncover the common, relevant food and nutrition concerns of the defined elderly, female, low-income population. Focus groups permit the researcher to hear the perceptions of participants without interjecting preconceived views. The respondents interact among themselves with minimal guidance. The facilitator merely leads the discussion along the desired route.

The four focus groups for this study were audio taped and partially transcribed. The typist recorded any segments in which the participants discussed potential barriers to healthful eating or expressed conerns. Content analysis revealed that the nutrition concerns of the participants could impact at the level of food acquisition, food preparation, or food consumption.

**Food Acquisition**

Problems with food acquisition result from transportation dilemmas and shopping difficulties. For the women who do not own a car or do not drive, a variety of transportation options are available, including Sr. Citizen buses, Dial-A-Ride, public buses, and friends or relatives. However, all of these options require some degree of planning ahead to utilize effectively. Furthermore, the elderly women stated that the public buses are difficult for disabled individuals to access. Even fully capable women complained of difficulty maneuvering bags of groceries onto and off the buses. One individual expressed her frustration:

> "I took the [*Dial-A-Ride*] bus once after I got home, to go shopping. You have to wait for them to come back and pick you up and I couldn't stand up very long for a period of time. So I only went that one time."

In general, the women who use the buses are very grateful for the service, although they do wish for more flexibility.

The gravest concern regarding grocery shopping is the high cost of food. Interestingly, the respondents expressed this issue as *"food costs too much,"* not *"we have too little money."* Cost constraints overlap and overshadow all other concerns. The *"end of the month"* is the most difficult period. Lorena[1] remained after one focus group to share her troubles.

> "I'd get what I could with what money I'd have and I've seen times when I didn't have it here too you know. But I went down to *[the community center]* and I cry when I think of it because I hate to think that I'm low like that. But, um, I went down to *[the community center]* and they gave me a bag of groceries and I got by. But now that I'm back on my feet a little bit, got my books straightened out, I have a freezer full of food, things like that and I get what I want. I shop once a month. (Pause). It's hard. I don't want to cry."

Stein et al. (1989) reported that older adults rated rising food costs as the most feared out of 37 potential stressors, including getting a fatal illness, becoming disabled, having to live in a nursing home, being robbed, or having to move. The researchers believed that their subjects viewed rising food costs as an immediate threat to survival.

Shopping concerns also include less alarming issues, such as food packaging and food quality. Purchase decisions include consideration of the weight of the item, the packaging material, and the portion size. Many focus participants agreed with Elsa's statement:

> "I wish they'd put bread out in smaller packages because I'd like to have different kinds of bread, you know, and get some rye bread, and you know, anything like that. But the great big loaves they have, they stay around forever. They get dried out. And I find that I waste bread. If they put out smaller packages of bread, then I could get different kinds."

The women also expressed worry over the quality of available foods. To some extent, the food quality issue is tied to the problem of financial constraints. Are the generic brands as good as the name brands? Is the day old produce as nutritious as the fresh produce? The complexity of food labels intensifies the concern over food quality.

Focus participants agreed that ingredient lists are difficult to read because of small print and mysterious ingredients, such as *"propylene glycol"* or *"disodium inosinate."* Furthermore, some women worried about the truthfulness of the labels.

## Food Preparation

Some women believe that *"It's a lot of bother to cook right."* Most of the participants cooked for their children and husbands for years and years. Now that they are alone, they sometimes lack the motivation to prepare a complete meal just for themselves.

> "It's not the same as when you're with family. You've got somebody to look forward to to sit down and eat with. You prepare enough you know. A lot of times because you're alone you don't feel like it."

The ease of meal preparation presented as a contradiction among the participants. On the one hand, they stated that they desire easy and quick cooking and cleanup. But simultaneously, capable individuals who did not prepare hot meals from scratch were considered *"lazy."*

> "A lot of people in here don't even cook."
>
> "They go out to eat rather than fix their own."
>
> "It's not because they can't."
>
> "Too lazy."

Heating up frozen dinners or eating cold meals indicates laziness. The women who follow these practices even label themselves as lazy. Interestingly, Howarth (1993) reported similar findings in her sample of 100 elders living in North London, England. The older adults defined a "proper meal" as consisting of hot foods including meat and two vegetables. Howarth (1993, 71) explained:

> The elderly women interviewed saw cooking as a task which transformed items of purchased food into something quite different. This conversion was achieved through a variety of processes including washing, chopping, slicing, seasoning, applying heat and

presentation. Using convenience foods was often not recognized by women as "proper cooking."

About one-half of the participants in this study also consider leftovers a problem. They stated that leftovers *"don't taste as good."* Packaging and storing leftovers is a hassle. In addition, some foods can not be kept for long periods, like tuna fish. The problem of leftovers is intensified since *"wasting food"* is viewed as morally wrong and financially foolish.

**Food Consumption**

Most women agreed that three meals a day are essential and that snacking is to be avoided. Snacking at night is especially viewed as taboo. However, the participants did vary in the degree to which they follow a mealtime routine. Some individuals appear highly regimented, eating the same foods at the same time everyday. For these women especially, changes in schedules caused by daily hassles and life stressors are likely to disorganize eating patterns.

Eating away from home is another instance when patterns must be altered. The participants believe that they should eat what is served when visiting friends or relatives. *"I eat what they give me on the table when I'm visiting, you know."* Similarly, less healthy foods are often available at social events. *"I go to Bingo Wednesday. I have a donut and coffee or something down there."* The women voiced more concern about what to do when offered foods cause them gastrointestinal distress, than when the foods are simply unhealthful. The conviction that they should eat what is served strictly holds when the food is high in fat, salt, or sugar. However, if the food is going to result in immediate physical distress, the item can be declined, but with some social awkwardness.

*Food Preferences*

Food preferences were discussed quite happily and at great length in all focus groups. Food likes and dislikes become a problem when they conflict with other nutrition messages creating discordance. For instance, Aileen, who had spoken earlier of high cholesterol, stated:

> "When I'm sick, I eat a dropped egg on toast. I think that makes the stomach feel so good."

While the dropped egg may be an emotionally comforting food, Aileen feels that she should limit the frequency she prepares it. Another frequent complaint was that food does not taste as good as it used to. When asked to specify which particular foods have changed in flavor, the women usually listed various cuts of meat and poultry.

## Modified diets

Modified diets can be differentiated between those that require certain foods to be included and those that require certain foods to be excluded. The two common reasons to include specific foods were bowel regularity and health promotion. Many participants follow an unwavering regime to avoid constipation. For example, Elaine rotates All Bran and Shredded Wheat every other day *"to keep me normal."* Health promoting foods include such items as olive oil, pasta, and cranberry juice.

The list of reasons to exclude foods and the number of foods that must be excluded is much longer than the list to include. Food and food constituents are excluded for health reasons, food allergies and insensitivities, weight loss efforts, and chewing difficulties.

The presence of chronic or degenerative diseases is most frequently the basis for limiting the intake of fat, salt, or sugar. The media appears to be the primary information source, although the physicians of some women have prescribed diets. The participants spoke of these health-related diet restrictions off and on throughout the entire discussion at all four focus groups. The need to limit certain foods was perceived as *"really a trial,"* as expressed by Lorna:

> "I never had diabetes before. It hit me a couple of years ago, that now I have to watch what I eat when I would like to eat everything in sight. It's really a trial. I had some grapes, but I actually can eat only 14. I'd like more than 14, but, you know, it's too much sugar. I count my grapes. I eat 14. I could eat a whole big *[large arm sweep]*. I love grapes."

Not following recommended diet restrictions was as frequently brought into the discussions as following them. *"I'm supposed to stay away from salt, but I usually cheat."*

Adverse gastrointestinal reactions and allergies also compel the women to avoid certain foods. These dietary restrictions are adhered to more strictly.

> "They say you are supposed to eat three and four vegetables and fruits a day. I couldn't do that. I'd be so sick, I wouldn't be able to, you know what I mean, my stomach like. Eggs, I can eat those probably once or twice a month, otherwise I'd be sick all the time. They don't agree with me."

The women identified snacking and sweets as the primary causes of being overweight. Thus many try to avoid these practices. Considering the advanced age of the participants, a relatively large number expressed an interest in weight loss.

Difficulty chewing certain foods also led to avoidance. The women specified red meat, raw or crisp-cooked vegetables, and nuts as the principal foods of concern. These foods are avoided in public situations, but not necessarily when eating at home, alone. Women with *"soft teeth"* avoided problem foods more consistently than women with dentures.

## Health

Health, both physical and mental, can impact at all levels – food acquisition, food preparation, and food consumption. The women referred to mental depression as being *"down in the dumps"* or *"worn out."* Feeling depressed can lead to over- or under-eating.

> *Mag:* You know something? If you don't feel good that has an awful lot to do with your diet. I mean, if you're worn out, you're going to snack. I found that out.
>
> *Stella:* If you're a bit down in the dumps, a bit depressed, you're less liable to eat good.
>
> *Mag:* When I'm down in the dumps, I eat.

*Vivian:* I'm just the opposite. When I'm upset, nervous, depressed, I can't eat. I can't sleep; I can't eat.

The women also discussed a *carpe diem* attitude that sometimes overrides cautions regarding cost or physical discomfort.

"I look at it this way, if I want something, I don't care what it costs."

"Well, that's what we should feel after all our struggle to reach the age we have."

The participants expressed more worry concerning the onset of acute illnesses than chronic disabilities. The focus groups consisted of women in stable situations that have most likely adapted to any existing functional incapability. Disabilities were spoken of as a constant annoyance that make all tasks more exhausting. *"Your arthritis kills you after you've carried a few heavy* [grocery] *bags."* Additional stressors are more difficult to overcome when disabilities are present.

In contrast, these women view acute illness as dire threats to well being. All of the participants live alone, and few have someone who would immediately jump in as caretaker. Food is stockpiled in case of such an emergency, as explained by Alice:

"You manage when you feel good and you can eat a lot. You put enough away in the fridge. So that when you don't care to eat you have something in the fridge you should eat."

Planning in advance is preferable, as illustrated by Gerta's remark:

"I'm gonna have a cataract removed, you know, an operation. And I'm going to prepare things I can easily take out of my refrigerator. Like I made chow mein. I'm preparing. And then I will have prepared food there in my refrigerator."

Acute illnesses take precedence and override other concerns. Frozen dinners are acceptable alternatives and gifts from friends are gladly accepted. Any special dietary constraints can be bent.

## Discussion

No new categories of nutrition concerns emerged after coding the first two focus sessions. The third and fourth sessions provided more illustrations and helped in interpretation of the findings. Thus, the repertoire of nutrition concerns appears fairly complete. A qualitative investigation by Falk, Bisogni, and Sobal (1996) further supports these results. They used in-depth interviewing techniques to uncover the food choice determinants in 16 older adults. While this analysis emphasized potential barriers to healthful eating and Falk, Bisogni, and Sobal (1996) considered all influences, the results are very similar.

Falk, Bisogni, and Sobal (1996) based their analysis on a food choice process model. They noted that the conviction *"that one eats whatever is served"* and childhood preferences exerted a large influence on the eating patterns of their informants. Finances and health were the next considerations. Similarly, cost and health appeared as the most universal concerns of the focus group participants in this study.

Food exclusions were the next most pressing concern, by the participants of both studies. However, as Falk, Bisogni, and Sobal (1996) also noted, food restrictions are common, but do not exert as great an impact on food selection as food preferences and ideals imprinted during childhood, finances, or health. Krondl et al. (1982) also investigated the food perceptions of elders. In their sample, taste preferences and health considerations guided food selection to a greater extent than price, convenience, or prestige (societal value).

## Issue Statements

The purpose of the focus groups was to delineate potential nutrition-related problems. Once potential problems were identified, the types of help offered in response to these problems could be ascertained in the key informant interviews.

Subsequently, the results extracted from the focus group discussions were condensed into 17 issue statements for use in the key informant interviews. (See Table 18.) Five follow-up interviews with prior focus group participants confirmed that the concepts and language of the issue statements were on-target and meaningful to this reference group. In addition, the follow-up interviews demonstrated that while the focus groups appeared to disclose the breadth of problems, personal interviews exposed the depth of the problems.

The 12 key informants further validated the relevance of the issue statements. The informants were familiar with all of the issues. During the in-depth interviews, informants discussed the types of help they receive in response to their top ranked concerns. Interestingly, the high cost of food was the most common concern. However, only one subject perceived any support in this area.

## HELPING BEHAVIORS

The primary purpose of the in-depth interviews was to discern the types of nutrition-related help perceived by elderly women. Previous research has examined the types of help perceived by low-income, young mothers (Gottlieb 1978), by caregivers of elderly parents (Abel 1989), and by cancer victims (Dakof and Taylor 1990). The generalizability of those results to a nutrition-specific situation with older women was unknown.

To uncover the types of nutrition-related help offered to the women in this study, the transcripts were coded following Gottlieb's (1978, 107) definition:

> The scoring unit consists of explicit descriptions of the helping behaviors — verbal, action-oriented, or material — which were extended and/or the qualities of the helper deemed influential. Statements describing the helper's impact on the respondent, frequently signaled by the stem, "X made me feel like . . ." were not acceptable as scoring units.

Only helping behaviors elicited in response to nutrition-related concerns were coded. For instance, the following passage was flagged as an example of help in acquiring groceries.

> "I have a license and everything, but at the place and time, I'm not driving. I went to the doctor's, and he said 'No, not for awhile.' This eye's degenerative, this one's got cataracts and narcoma. So my two daughters do the grocery shopping, and my aide will, if I need something."

**Table 18: Individuals who ranked each concern as a major concern in their life, discussed the concern in detail during the interview, or ranked the concern as applicable (major or minor concern in their life)**

| Concern | Key Informants (n=12) | | All [a] (n=17) |
|---|---|---|---|
| | Major Concern | Discussed in Detail | Applicable |
| I don't drive to the grocery store. | 9 | 6 | 11 |
| These days, food costs too much. | 8 | 1 | 16 |
| I have to watch my diet. | 7 | 7 | 12 |
| Shopping and cooking are difficult because of my disabilities. | 6 | 9 | 10 |
| When I'm down in the dumps I don't eat right. | 6 | 4 | 11 |
| I am working to lose weight. | 5 | 3 | 12 |
| They don't sell foods in the small portion sizes I need. | 5 | 2 | 11 |
| Grocery shopping is tiring. | 5 | 1 | 11 |
| Sometimes I don't feel like going to all the bother of cooking just for myself. | 5 | 1 | 10 |
| I eat certain foods to avoid constipation. | 5 | 0 | 10 |
| When I'm sick I don't cook. | 4 | 2 | 12 |
| Some foods don't agree with me. | 4 | 1 | 8 |
| Foods don't taste as good as they did in the past. | 4 | 1 | 8 |
| I snack too much at night. | 3 | 1 | 3 |
| I forget to eat meals. | 2 | 0 | 2 |
| When I eat away from home, I eat foods that I shouldn't. | 1 | 0 | 10 |
| Some foods take too much effort to chew. | 0 | 0 | 5 |

[a] The results for applicability include the 12 key informants plus the five focus group follow-up recruits.

The descriptions of helping behaviors were then grouped and categorized. Table 19 outlines a schema of the most frequently discussed helping behaviors. At least three examples of each of these helping behaviors were described by at least two key informants. Many examples of instrumental help and availability were expressed. Fewer instances of informational and emotional help were recounted.

**Table 19: Schema of common nutrition-related helping behaviors in response to two identified stressors: food acquisition and modified diets**

I. Instrumental Help
    A. Food preparation
    B. Grocery shopping
    C. Drives
    D. Accompanies
II. Availability
III. Informational
    A. Direction
    B. Advice
    C. Education
IV. Emotional
    A. Encouragement
    B. Self-disclosure

**Instrumental**

The instrumental helping behaviors are mainly elicited in response to poor health or physical limitations. Most of the instrumental help is for the purpose of food acquisition. Some women in this age group have never driven. They remain dependent on others for transportation. *"My daughter and I go shopping together. I don't get out any other way myself."*

Food preparation refers to a spectrum of activities ranging from preparing entire, well-balanced meals to repackaging foods for storage and later use. Laura has painful, rheumatoid arthritis and has been blind for many years. Her lack of sight and limited finger dexterity make cooking almost impossible. She attends congregate meals a few times each week and her three daughters assist her on the weekends. Laura explained, *"I manage somehow to cook most days. But it's awful nice to have the meals cooked over the weekend."* Her daughters also help her with partial food preparation.

> "She takes my hamburg and she divides it in four sections and puts it all in aluminum foil. You could open the top of my refrigerator and you'd see it there the way she fixes it."

Because her daughter has packaged her food in individual portions, Laura can prepare her own dinner whenever she does not like the congregate menu.

Similarly, grocery shopping refers to a spectrum ranging from purchase of all foods needed by the recipient to an occasional pick-up of milk or orange juice. Irene, an 81-year-old women with diabetes, explained:

> "My youngest daughter, Marilyn, she does my food shopping every Tuesday. I mark down whatever I need, and then she calls me up, she writes it down, and then she goes and picks it up and brings it home. She's been doing this for 17 years, after my husband had Parkinson's because I've never learned to drive. I've got good girls you know; they're good to me."

Thelma's daughter also does her grocery shopping each week. In addition, Thelma has an aide. She stated, *"I run short on something, milk or something, the aide will run up and get it."*

Accompaniment is a precautionary measure. Carol, a 79-year-old widow with mildly impaired functional status, explained her reliance on her friend.

> "As a rule, I go with my friend, Flo. I'd like to go by myself, but, I'm afraid. I get a cart right in front of my car. Generally, somebody leaves a cart there. And that's what my brace is. I have a cane, but how do you manage a cane, and your cart and your groceries and everything else? So, I go with Flo. We go our separate ways, but, we wait for each other. If she's at the cashier before I am, she waits for me. She's the one."

## Availability

The availability and accessibility of helpers is very important to the informants. Comments such as *"She's always there"* or *"He's always willing to help"* were repeatedly used to describe key sources of support. Typically the informants raised the issue of accessibility when discussing the providers of instrumental aid. For instance, in the example above, Carol continued with appreciation for her fellow tenant.

> "Flo's a sweetheart. She's always willing to help. This morning she's taking a man to the doctor, this afternoon she's taking me to get my car washed and to the grocery store. She's just available, she's just there, you know. She's always willing to help."

## Informational

Providers typically offer informational types of help in response to special diet needs. Directive behaviors are those that spell out what the recipient should do. Health professionals directed Mary to follow an exchange plan. *"Of course, when the diabetes came along, they decided to put me on the ADA diet, no salt, and that's on all of it."* Providers of directive help also enforce the dietary restrictions. The elderly women view these instances of help as positive behaviors. For example, Irene, the 81-year-old widow with diabetes, explained how her two daughters monitor her diet.

> "My daughter said, 'Make sure Ma you don't cheat now'. I said, 'You can ask anyone that is at *[the congregate meal]* if I cheat, you can ask them. They'll tell you I don't cheat.' My daughters are very concerned about me."

Similarly, sources of support offer advice or suggestions to help the informants follow their diets. Advice infers that the recipient has a choice, although the predilection of the provider is evident. Thelma, who suffers with lactose intolerance, described the suggestion of her physician.

"He told me that it would be a good idea. It would help me since I had that problem with the diarrhea. I can get that very easy. And so he thought it would be a good idea if I took that nutrition class. If I wanted to. I didn't have to. But I did."

Education implies even more choice on the part of the recipient. For example, a Registered Dietitian explained a prescribed 1500–calorie diet to Gladys, a 76-year-old widow with diabetes. Gladys disagreed with her physician's orders. She felt that 1500 calories was too high. Instead, she decided to restrict herself to 1200 calories. She considered the dietitian's information helpful when amending her diet plan.

"I can't eat 1500 calories. It's too much, too much. So I just go my own way. I thought I was eating too much meat, but according to what she said, I should be eating more. She straightened me out, about my bread, about my meat."

A second example is Lois's physician who provided education regarding weight loss.

"What he did, he said to me, 'Well, if you want I'll give you, like um, not a diet, but information on foods that you could eliminate.' He said, 'If you think losing weight is important, this might help you'."

**Emotional**

The informants also discussed two types of emotionally supportive behaviors in response to modified diets. Encouragement refers to behaviors that bolster the confidence of the participants and reassure them of the importance of their diets. Helen monitors the salt in her diet. Her doctor told her *"Well, you're doing the right thing; do it the way you are doing it."* Irene, the widow with diabetes mentioned above, explained how her daughters provide encouragement.

"I still weigh my food sometimes, like when I see that the chicken's got a bigger leg or something, I'll weigh it. My daughters say 'That's important when you're a diabetic with insulin'."

Self-disclosure refers to the sharing of a similar situation, without undertones of advice or judgment. Selma explained the conversations with her friend. *"It helps to talk back with her, 'cause I tell her about what we can have, sugar patients, and she tells me what she's doing."* Lois, an energetic 80-year-old, discussed how her friend has aided her during a three-year effort to lose weight.

"There are quite a few here that have a weight, I don't know if you want to call it a problem or, but they are aware of their weight. They'll be passing around little pieces of cake and coffee and Sue'll say, 'I'd better not have any of that today'. I say, 'Oh, you can't have that?' She says, 'No, I can't seem to get this weight off' .... We talk about how we feel. I think we make each other feel better."

**Other**

The analyses did reveal one or two instances of further types of nutrition-related support. Only one key informant described each of these types of help.

- Referral for additional help: The helper files an authorized referral for a service such as Meals-on-Wheels or a Dietitian consult.
- Distraction from the situation: The helper changes the topic of conversation to other, positive aspects of life, or takes the respondent out for an enjoyable time to take her mind off worries.
- Reflecting deep understanding: The helper expresses total empathy with the situation of the respondent, such as the necessity of following a restrictive, therapeutic diet.
- Role-modeling: The helper provides an example of successful coping that the respondent tries to emulate, such as taking the time and initiative to prepare healthful meals for *a single person.*

# Nutrition-Related Concerns and Proffered Help

In addition, the informants described numerous instances of oversupport and undersupport. Oversupport are instances where helping behaviors become controlling. While Gladys usually considers her daughter helpful, sometimes her daughter goes overboard. Gladys explained:

> "She's the mother and I'm the daughter now. So it seems. She listens to the doctor, she knows what the doctor, the doctors explain things to her then she explains them to me. As though I can't hear or something. . . . She wants me to lose weight. She insists that I eat a lot of fats. And I can't see where I eat a lot of fats. . . . She keeps at me all the time."

Oversupport also occurs when network members perceive a problem that the focal individual does not recognize. Marge described her son as a *"health nut."* She does not interpret his advice or gifts of healthy food as supportive.

> "So I was telling my son about *[new frozen dinners on the market]*, and he said 'Ma, don't eat those things, they're too fat for you!' I said, 'Tom, at this late date, why am I worrying over that now'?"

Undersupport refers to occasions when help is not offered or is perceived as insufficient. Undersupport often occurs when network members are unaware of an adverse situation, or interpret the situation as less threatening than the focal individual. Angie is a moderately overweight, active 77-year-old woman, recently diagnosed with hypertension. Her physician prescribed a low sodium diet. Photos on Angie's table show an overweight family. Her children and grandchildren are convinced that Angie's recent weight loss signifies poor health. Angie described the reaction at a holiday meal where none of the foods traditionally served met her new dietary needs.

> "They'll beg me to eat one little, 'Look at how skinny you're getting'. They're not thinking of my blood pressure. They're not even thinking of my blood pressure, you know. They'll just tell me to eat. 'Grandma, look at how skinny you are.' They can't believe that I

shouldn't eat. The way I used to eat before, they can't believe the way I eat now."

Some of the informants reported that no one was available for support in response to a particular concern. *"I'm on my own."* Others believe they should not reveal certain problems. Thus, support is not activated.

"I wouldn't talk like that, to anybody, I'm telling you *[about my problem with diverticulitis]*, here, now, but I wouldn't go around telling it to everybody else. Maybe I would tell the doctor, if he asks."

The definition of social support for this project *only included behaviors that were perceived as helpful.* Instances of oversupport and undersupport were carefully excluded from the categorization schema. Their existence is briefly mentioned here to emphasize the importance of fully understanding the perceptions of the support recipient. Distinguishing between directing and controlling behaviors is particularly difficult, as well as identifying support attempts that are perceived as insufficient.

## CONCLUSION

The focus groups permitted identification of common food and nutrition problems as perceived by elderly women. The concerns were condensed into 17 issue statements for use in the key informant interviews. The high cost of food was the most common concern. The women also expressed concern about transportation to the grocery store, modified diets, and difficulty cooking and shopping due to disabilities.

Analyses of the twelve key informant interviews revealed that the majority of the nutrition-related helping behaviors could be classified into four categories, with a total of 10 types of help. Furthermore, almost all of the helping behaviors were elicited in response to two problems: physical limitations and diet modifications.

The types of helping behaviors appear somewhat similar to those found by Gottlieb (1978) in his study of low-income, young mothers. He documented a greater variety of helping behaviors and developed a slightly different classification scheme. The young mothers perceive more nondirective types of aid, such as unfocused talking and listening, and fewer controlling types of aid. The differences could result from characteristics of the samples as well as differences in the problems facing these two groups.

Similarly, the helping behaviors reported by the elderly women in this study are similar to many of the types of help extended to filial caregivers (Abel 1989) and to cancer victims (Dakof and Taylor 1990). For instance, the respondents in all of the studies (the young mothers, the caregivers, the cancer victims, and the elderly women of this study) noted receipt of advice and self-disclosure.

However, discrepancies also exist between the types of aid offered to the groups. For example, only the caregivers mentioned sibling help with decision making; only the cancer victims described physical presence (just being there); only the young mothers recounted buffering (preventing contact between mother and stressor). The differences are not surprising considering the particulars of each study. Clearly, social support is a complex phenomena specific to the situation (Cohen and Wills 1985) and to the interpersonal relationships involved in the situation.

Phase II of this project was designed to further explore the details of nutrition-related help. The Nutrition Social Support Questionnaire was developed based on the helping behavior schema described above. The following chapter discusses the frequency and the providers of nutrition-related social support reported by the larger sample of 102 participants.

**NOTES**

1. Names of participants have been changed throughout this book to protect anonymity.

CHAPTER 5
# Nutrition-Related Social Support

The first objective of this research study was to develop a classification schema of the functions of nutrition-related social support, presented in the previous chapter. The next objective was to examine the types and providers of nutrition support in a larger sample. A third objective was to describe the satisfaction of the respondents with the provision and providers of nutrition support.

To meet these objectives, 102 elderly women were interviewed about the types of help they receive with food consumption, food acquisition, and food preparation. The results of the focus groups and key informant interviews had demonstrated that the need for diet modifications was a significant source of stress affecting food consumption. Thus, help with modified diets was operationally defined as *"help following a special diet or eating in a more healthful way."* The qualitative results indicated that emotional and informational types of support may be offered in response to the stresses of modified diets.

The providers and types of help with food acquisition and food preparation were also investigated in the larger sample. Help with food acquisition was operationally defined as *"help with obtaining groceries."* Help with food preparation was defined as *"help with preparing meals or obtaining prepared meals."* The qualitative exploration revealed that respondents receive instrumental types of aid for the purposes of food acquisition and food preparation. Thus, the results for food acquisition and preparation are discussed simultaneously under food and meal procurement.

In this chapter, the types and providers of help are discussed in detail. Both informal and formal sources of support are considered. The satisfaction of the respondents with proffered support is explored. In addition, the strengths and weaknesses of the support system are examined in conjunction with previously published work.

## MODIFIED DIETS

An older adult with a chronic condition, such as diabetes or hypertension, can often maximize health by following a therapeutic diet. The individual's physician is most likely to prescribe the appropriate diet, for instance a diabetic exchange plan for a senior with diabetes. In addition, many older adults today are following preventative diets. An individual with a family history of coronary artery disease may personally decide to eat a diet low in fat.

However, changing an eating pattern is rarely easy. Dietary habits can become deeply ingrained over the course of a lifetime. Heritage, financial resources, food preferences, health attitudes, educational opportunities, and many other factors intertwine to influence the ultimate diet. An older adult who decides to change her food patterns must be informed about the reality of how to implement the changes. Simultaneously, she must change some of her food traditions, attitudes and beliefs.

The functions of social support are to supply the knowledge and encouragement the purposeful recipient needs for success. Respondents in this study noted that both informational and emotional support are offered to aid them in improving their diets. For instance, in a best case scenario, a physician prescribes a low sodium diet for an elderly patient, Marge. The doctor then refers Marge to a dietitian for further instruction. Marge's daughter accompanies her so that she can help by purchasing appropriate foods and providing encouragement for her mother. Follow-up visits with the dietitian are conducted for continued learning. Other family members and friends bolster Marge's efforts by offering suggestions, reassurance and additional forms of support.

### Physician- and Self-prescribed Diets

In this study, 94% of the subjects report following a modified diet. Most adhere to multiple restrictions. Table 20 shows the number of physician- and self-prescribed diets that the women follow. On average, these subjects juggle the requirements of $2^1/_2$ diets. Approximately one-third follow only physician-prescribed diets, one-third follow only self-prescribed diets, and one-third follow a mixture of physician- and self-prescribed diets.

Table 20: Physician- and self-prescribed modified diets

|  | Physician-prescribed (n=60) | | Self-prescribed (n=70) | | Combined (n=96 [a]) | |
|---|---|---|---|---|---|---|
|  | n | % | n | % | n | % |
| Number of Modifications |  |  |  |  |  |  |
| 1 | 29 | 48 | 32 | 46 | 27 | 28 |
| 2 | 16 | 27 | 26 | 37 | 29 | 30 |
| 3 | 8 | 13 | 8 | 11 | 16 | 17 |
| 4 | 5 | 8 | 3 | 4 | 17 | 18 |
| 5 or more | 2 | 3 | 1 | 1 | 7 | 7 |
| Type of Modification |  |  |  |  |  |  |
| Low fat | 27 | 47 | 28 | 41 | 55 | 57 |
| Avoid irritants [b] | 10 | 17 | 31 | 46 | 41 | 43 |
| Low sodium | 26 | 45 | 12 | 18 | 38 | 40 |
| Low cholesterol | 21 | 36 | 11 | 16 | 32 | 33 |
| Low sugar | 6 | 10 | 14 | 21 | 20 | 21 |
| Weight loss | 10 | 17 | 3 | 4 | 13 | 14 |
| More fruit & veg. | 0 | 0 | 11 | 16 | 11 | 11 |
| More calcium | 0 | 0 | 4 | 6 | 4 | 4 |
| High fiber | 1 | 2 | 3 | 4 | 4 | 4 |
| Diabetic | 3 | 5 | 0 | 0 | 3 | 3 |
| Lactose free | 1 | 2 | 2 | 3 | 3 | 3 |
| Low fiber | 3 | 5 | 0 | 0 | 3 | 3 |
| Low starch | 1 | 2 | 2 | 3 | 3 | 3 |
| Weight gain | 2 | 3 | 0 | 0 | 2 | 2 |
| Bland | 2 | 3 | 0 | 0 | 2 | 2 |
| Other [c] | 2 | 3 | 4 | 6 | 6 | 6 |
| Total Types | 115 | 100 | 125 | 100 | 240 | 100 |

[a] Total study n=102; only 6 participants reported no special diet considerations.
[b] The avoidance of specific foods due to diverticulosis, gastroesophageal reflux, food allergies and insensitivities.
[c] Includes one instance each: low iron, decrease snacks, decrease processed foods, no oxalates, high iron, and no seafood due to contaminants.

Table 20 further shows the variety of diets as described by the women in this study. The most common diet is a low fat regime mentioned by over one-half of the subjects. The low sodium diet appears to originate more often from physicians than from subjects. Subjects appear more concerned with avoiding irritating foods than do their physicians.

The diets that these women report following are not always appropriate nor well understood by them. For instance, one individual who experienced gestational diabetes 60 years prior continues to eat a low starch diet per her doctor's recommendation in the 1930's. The infrequent mention of high fiber, which would benefit a large proportion of these subjects, is another example of insufficient dietary guidance.

## Diet Support

Over three-quarters of the subjects feel that their diets are very important and state that they follow them most of the time. But only 40 of the 96 women believe that they have received any support in the past year for their efforts. Women on physician-prescribed diets are more likely to receive support than women on self-prescribed diets ($\chi^2$=6.58, p<.01, $df$=1). Following a greater number of modifications does not increase the likelihood of support ($\chi^2$=7.01, p=.14, $df$=4). Correlation analyses showed no statistically significant associations between the likelihood of diet support and demographic, health, or social variables (including age, education, rent, health, years alone, years at complex, functional status, BMI, social anchorage, overall help received, or reciprocal help).

### Providers of Diet Support

Figure 4 shows the number of helpers per respondent. Most subjects report no help within the past year. Of those who have received diet support, over one-half cite only one helper. Even though the diet needs of many of these subjects are quite complex, less than one in five perceive diet support from more than one person. For women who do receive support, the number of helpers is similar whether the diet was physician-prescribed or self-prescribed (analysis of variance for an unbalanced design [PROC GLM] p=.70).

**Figure 4: Size of diet support networks of 96 elderly women who report following modified diets**

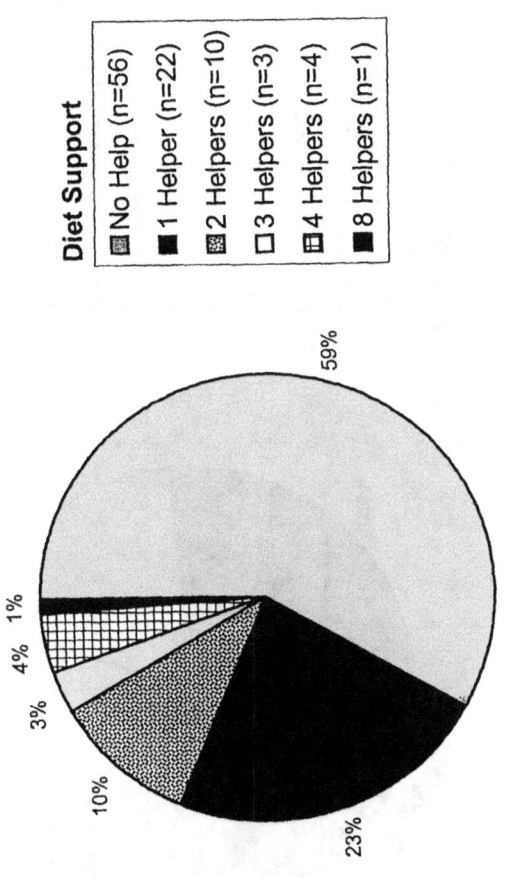

**Figure 5: Relationship of diet support providers (n=75) to respondents (n=40)**

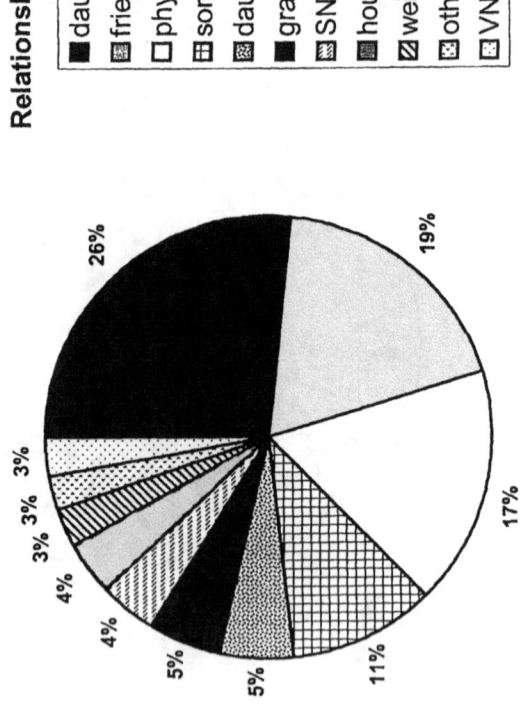

A total of 75 individuals provide diet support to the subjects in this study. Figure 5 shows the relationships of the helpers to the respondents. The primary sources of support are daughters, friends, and physicians, accounting for almost two-thirds of all helpers. Interestingly, three subjects mentioned Senior Nutrition Awareness Project staff. In four instances the interviews occurred after the nutrition education program had been implemented. Three out of those four individuals noted the positive influence of SNAP staff. Other than SNAP staff and perhaps weight loss group leaders, no mention of nutritionists or dietitians was made.

*Types of Diet Support*

The key informant interviews of Phase I indicated that diet help to older adults is mainly in the forms of informational and emotional support. In agreement with the findings from Phase I, the most common types of help reported in the second phase include advice, encouragement, education, direction, and self-disclosure. Almost one-half to three-quarters of the respondents who receive aid report each of these types. Figure 6 shows the number of respondents who secure each form of support from at least one provider.

Women who follow only self-prescribed diets receive significantly less encouragement than do women on physician-prescribed diets ($\chi^2=9.21$, $p=.01$, $df=2$). Although the differences are not statistically different, they also appear to receive less education, directives, and advice than do women following physician-prescribed diets.

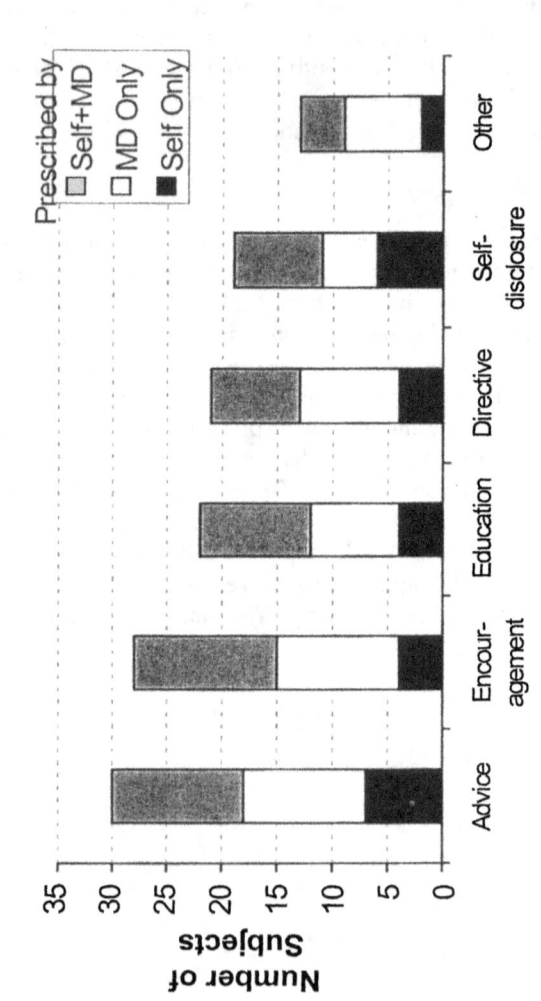

**Figure 6: Number of subjects receiving each type of support by origin of diet**

NOTE: Forty out of the 96 women following modified diets reported receiving at least one type of help.
Advice = suggestions on how to follow diet guidelines.
Encouragement = reassurance and motivation to follow diet.
Education = diet instruction and counseling.
Directive = firm guidance and monitoring of diet.
Self-disclosure = sharing of similar diet situation, without undertones of advice or judgment.
Other = 10 instances of acknowledgement of modified diets and one instance each of role modeling, empathy, and referral.
(See Chapter 4 for further descriptions and examples.)

Figure 6 shows 13 women who reported other types of help in following their diets. Ten of the cases in this category refer to acknowledgment of modified diets through the provision of appropriate foods. The affirmation of their dietary restrictions, which is a form of emotional support, appears more important to the respondents than the contribution of food, a type of instrumental aid. The three other cases refer to one instance each of role modeling, empathy, and referral.

## Provider-Type Specificity

Table 21 shows the specifics of which providers supply each type of diet support. In this study, daughters are by far the greatest sources of diet support to their elderly mothers. Not only do daughters supply the greatest total types of help, they also furnish more types of help per provider. On average, daughters contribute slightly over three types of support, in contrast to slightly over two types of support for sons, and slightly under two types of support for friends or for physicians.

Daughters offer the most advice and, along with sons, the most encouragement. Daughters also offer the most diet education, notably more than physicians. Physicians, daughters, and sons all offer a fair number of directive behaviors. Friends are noted for their distinctive contribution of self-disclosure.

**Table 21: Diet support providers and types of support**

| Type of Support[a] | Daughters (n=20) | Friends (n=14) | Physicians (n=13) | Sons (n=8) |
|---|---|---|---|---|
| Advice | 15 | 4 | 4 | 3 |
| Affirmation | 4 | 4 | 0 | 2 |
| Directive | 9 | 0 | 7 | 4 |
| Education | 11 | 2 | 5 | 1 |
| Encouragement | 17 | 6 | 7 | 8 |
| Self-disclosure | 7 | 11 | 1 | 0 |
| Total | 63 | 27 | 24 | 18 |
| Types/Provider | 3.2 | 1.9 | 1.8 | 2.3 |

[a] See Figure 6 for a description of the types of help.

Table 21 includes 70% of the diet help perceived by the respondents. The remaining 30% of the help is received from an additional 20 individuals representing seven relationship categories. The number in each relationship category is too small to draw conclusions. However, of consideration is the helping profile of the four daughters-in-law. The types and amount of help they offer is similar to that of daughters.

**Satisfaction with Diet Support**

The majority of subjects stated that they are satisfied with the diet support they receive. Only 18 of the 96 individuals following a modified diet indicated that they would prefer more support. One-half of the women who desire more support are currently receiving no support; the other one-half already receive some emotional or informational aid. Figure 7 shows the types of additional help these women would like.

The associations between wanting more diet support and demographic, health, and social variables were examined through correlation analyses. The specific variables included age, education, rent, self-rated health, number of years lived alone, number of years in present complex, functional status, BMI, social anchorage, total number of individuals who provide general support, and total number of individuals for whom subject provides support (reciprocal support).

The only variable related to wanting support for women who do not currently receive aid is the number of years they have lived alone (Spearman r= -.33, p=.02). On average, women who want support have lived alone only 14 years, while women who feel that support is not needed have lived alone 24 years.

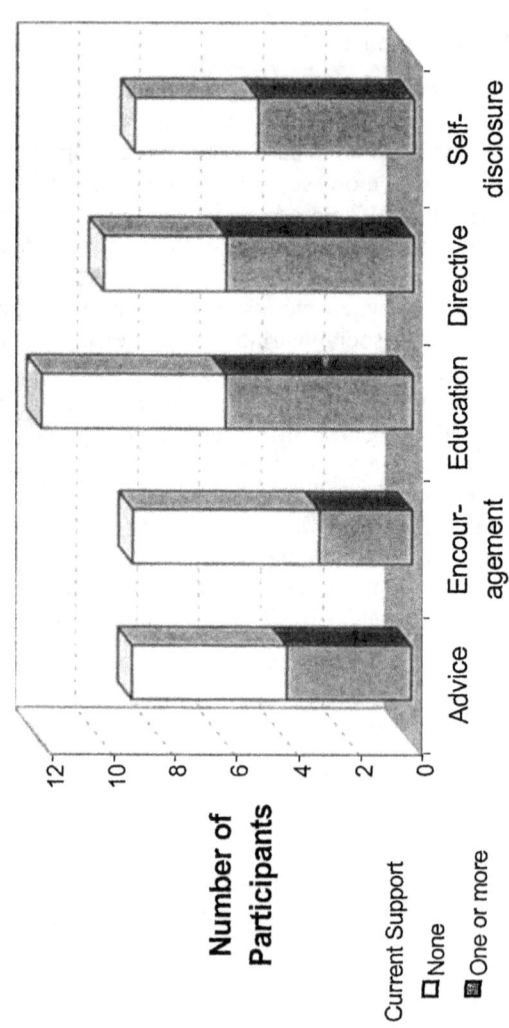

**Figure 7:** Types of help that subjects feel would benefit their diet efforts (n=18). See Figure 6 for a description of the types of help.

For women already receiving some diet support, age (Spearman r=-.40, p=.01) and BMI (Spearman r=.40, p=.01) are related to wanting more support. That is, women who would like more support are significantly younger and heavier. For the entire group of women, both those currently receiving support and those not currently receiving support, BMI is also significantly related to the belief that one or more individuals has tried to help them, but that the help was ineffectual (Spearman r=-.33, p=.001).

**Table 22: Women currently receiving diet support—comparison between those who want more support and those who are satisfied**

|  | Want more support (n=9) | Satisfied with support (n=30) |
|---|---|---|
| Number of Helpers |  |  |
| 1 | 4 | 17 |
| 2 | 3 | 7 |
| 3 | 0 | 3 |
| 4 | 1 | 3 |
| 8 | 1 | 0 |
| Primary Providers [a] |  |  |
| Friends | 6 | 8 |
| Daughters | 4 | 16 |
| Sons | 4 | 4 |
| Physicians | 2 | 11 |
| Types of Help [b] |  |  |
| Advice | 6 | 23 |
| Encouragement | 7 | 20 |
| Education | 6 | 15 |
| Directive | 4 | 16 |
| Self-disclosure | 4 | 15 |

NOTE: Total n=40. Information missing for one subject.
[a] Many individuals receive help from more than one source. Thus total of columns may be greater than total n.
[b] See Figure 6 for a description of the types of help. Most individuals receive more than one type of help, thus total of column may be greater than total n.

One objective of this study was to examine the association between satisfaction with support and the types and providers of support. Certain types of help or certain providers of help might be perceived as more satisfactory than other types of help or other providers of help.

However, the number of women who are currently receiving support but wish for more is too small in this sample to draw any conclusions (n=9). No obvious differences are apparent between those who desire more support and those who are satisfied with the present level of support in the number of support providers, the relationships of the support providers, or types of help received. Table 22 shows a comparison between the two groups.

## Discussion

A full 94% of the women in this study follow modified diets, either physician- or self-prescribed. Other researchers have reported lower incidences of modified diets (Table 23). The questionnaire wording, broad definition of "modified diet," and characteristics of the sample most likely led to the high incidence.

**Table 23: Incidence of modified diets in related literature and this study**

| Research Group | Sample Characteristics | Diet (%) | | |
| --- | --- | --- | --- | --- |
| | | Physician-Prescribed | Self-Prescribed | Total |
| This study | 102 F 75–95 years | 58 | 68 | 96 |
| LeClerc-1983 | 53 M+F 60+ years | 47 | | |
| Lee-1993 | 3,021 M+F 65–106 years | | | 44 |
| Shifflett-1986 | 165 F elderly | | | 47 |
| Westenbrink-1989 | 369 F 65–79 | 33 | | |

On average the women in this study concurrently balance $2^1/_2$ types of dietary restrictions, most commonly low fat, low sodium, and avoiding irritating foods. Following dietary constraints while continuing to eat a variety of foods is important to achieve maximum health, but is often a complicated issue. Furthermore, some of the dietary restrictions these women follow appear unfounded. The complexity of the diet is increased without additional health benefits.

Although their diets are often intricate and are vital for optimal health, most of the women in this study perceive no support in their efforts to follow the restrictions. One subject stated that she no longer has dinner at a good friend's house, because the friend continues to serve high fat meats the subject should not eat. Another respondent wondered why her children continue to bring her gifts of chocolate candy when they can clearly see that her obesity is compromising her health.

Only 40 women perceive support in following their diets. Subjects who follow at least one physician-prescribed diet have an increased likelihood of receiving support. Women following self-prescribed diets receive notably less encouragement, and perhaps less advice, education, and direction. The physician intervention is an indicator of supportive actions—perhaps tied to perceived credibility of the diet or importance of the diet.

Daughters are the largest source of support, accounting for almost one-third of the total help received. Daughters are major providers of advice, encouragement, and education. Friends offer self-disclosure, a notably low form of help from daughters. Physicians, the other significant providers of diet support, are most likely to supply encouragement and directives.

Toner (1987) also found that older adults enrolled in a nutrition workshop reported low levels of nutrition and diet support. The workshop subjects perceived more help from family and friends than health professionals. However, support from neither group was strong.

The low incidence of diet support raises concern. Could it be possible that elderly women do not recognize offers of diet support? Or could it be that they refuse overtures of help? Many respondents in this study expressed sentiments such as *"the motivation needs to come from within"* and *"nobody can do it but you yourself."* Furthermore, only a small number believed that they might benefit from increased levels of support. Abel (1989), in her study of caregivers of elderly parents, noted that her informants seemed hesitant to discuss emotionally sustaining types of support. These findings suggest that emotional independence is important to this cohort. Thus, diet support needs to be presented as a tool for continued empowerment, not as a crutch for the needy.

## FOOD AND MEAL PROCUREMENT

In order to maintain an independent living situation, individuals must be able to obtain and prepare food. Older adults may find these tasks challenging for a number of reasons such as poor stamina, the inability to drive, arthritis, or other physical and functional limitations. Both formal and informal sources of support exist to help elders meet their shopping and cooking needs. Examples of formal services include senior bus lines, homemaker agencies, grocery delivery, and home delivered meals. Friends and relatives may provide equivalent services or they may supplement the formal system.

### Case Descriptions

The following two case studies contrast the situations of Josephine and Evelyn. Both widows have numerous physical and functional limitations. However, Josephine has taken advantage of a variety of nutrition support options. In comparison, Evelyn relies on only one source of help.

Josephine is a 91-year-old widow. She is legally blind, has chronic bronchitis, and is wheelchair-bound when outside her apartment. Her functional status is rated severely impaired. Although a physician has never prescribed a modified diet, she is very nutrition conscious. She eliminated pork and shellfish from her diet over 60 years ago because of religious beliefs. She also eliminated dairy and nuts due to severe allergic reactions.

Josephine has only lived in her present apartment for five years, yet she is well embedded in a nutrition support system. She receives Meals-on-Wheels three days each week and rides the Senior bus to a local congregate meal site twice a week. Her son does her major grocery shopping once a month. These groceries are supplemented by both her daughter, who picks up items every other week, and her homemaker, who shops for her each week. Both her daughter and a friend drop by with gifts of food, such as soup and home-baked bread, a few times each month. Josephine limits her breakfast and dinner to foods that she considers both healthful and easy to prepare.

Evelyn is also a widow, but is 15 years younger than Josephine. She has hypertension, arthritis, aortic stenosis and phlebitis; all presumably complicated by her obesity (BMI = 43.5). Her functional

## Nutrition-Related Social Support

status is moderately impaired. Evelyn's physician recommended a low fat, low sugar diet that she feels is somewhat important. She also needs to avoid foods that give her heartburn.

Evelyn is unable to shop. She does not receive any formal sources of nutrition support. Instead she pays a friend to shop and clean for her once a week. No one else picks up groceries, nor shares food with her. Evelyn never attends the meal programs at her apartment complex. She stated, *"If it weren't for Patches* [her pet cat], *I wouldn't even bother to cook."*

### Obtaining Groceries

While Evelyn and Josephine have contrasting levels of service use, they are both totally dependent on others to provide them with groceries. At the other extreme are the totally self-reliant women who participated in this study. They complete all their own shopping, without ever asking one friend to pick up a quart of orange juice or a box of Corn Flakes. Figure 8 shows the spectrum of aid that the women in this study receive in acquiring their groceries. (The abbreviations are used in Figure 9.)

**Figure 8: Ascending levels of support in acquiring groceries**

A. None *(none)*
B. Occasional pick up of small items *(pick-up)*
C. Transportation *(trans)*
D. Transportation + "B" *(trans + pick-up)*
E. Occasional accompaniment for health/safety reasons + "D" *(occ accomp)*
F. Accompaniment for health/safety reasons, always + "D" *(always accomp)*
G. Provides all groceries *(all shopping)*

As would be expected, the types of support vary with the functional status of the subject. Figure 9 shows the types of help in acquiring groceries in relation to functional status. In general, women with greater functional limitations report receiving higher levels of support than women with fewer functional limitations. Of concern are the exceptions. Note the two moderately impaired women who receive no help. Are they able to obtain all the food they need?

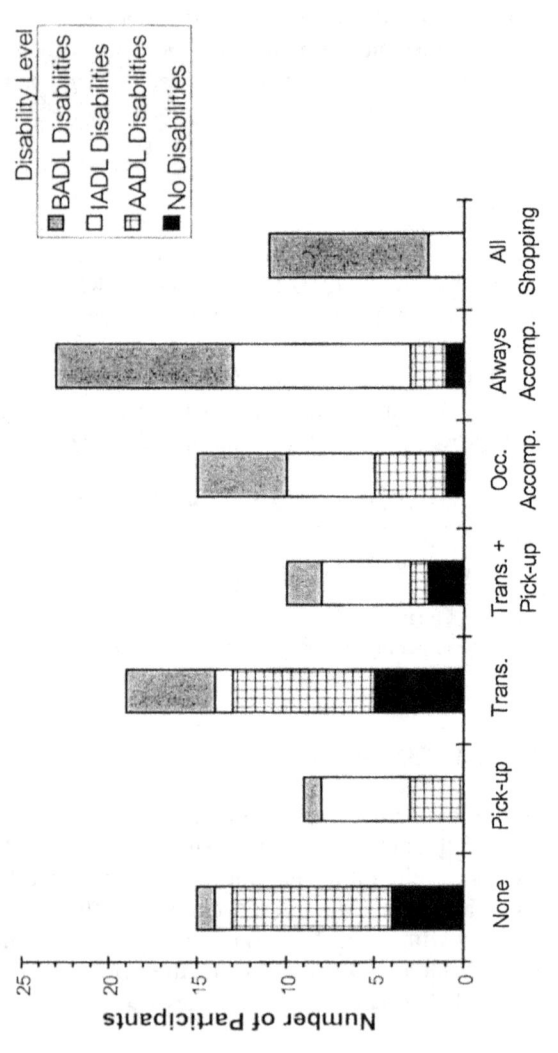

Figure 9: Support in acquiring groceries by functional status. See Figure 8 for a further description of the types of support.

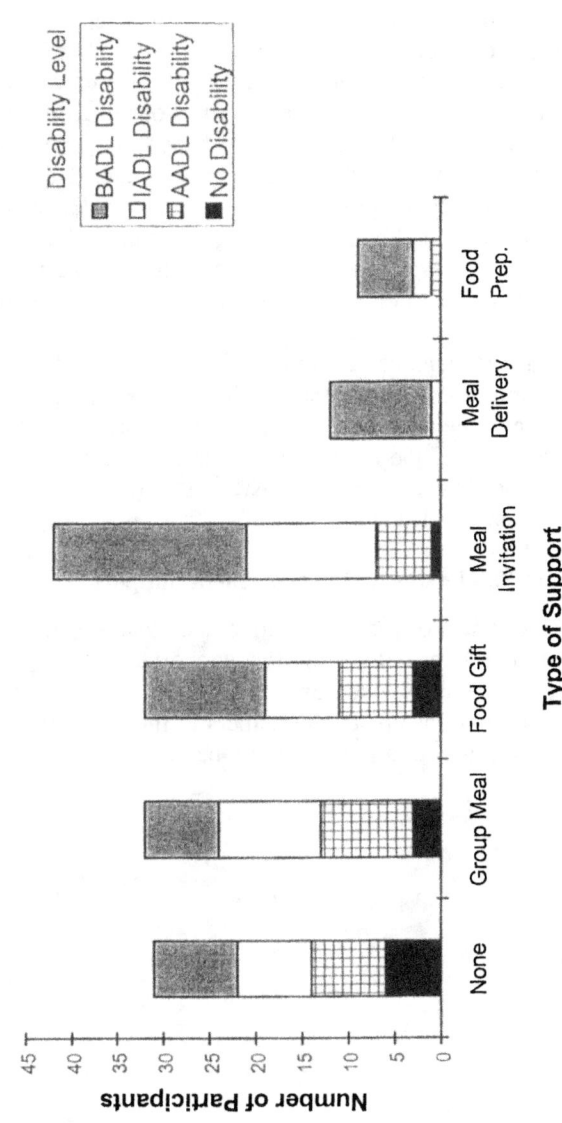

Figure 10: Support in acquiring meals by functional status

*Obtaining Meals*

Either groceries must be transformed into a meal, or a ready prepared meal may be obtained. The women in this study report five types of help in this area: help with food preparation, gifts of food, home delivered meals, group meals, and invitations to a meal. Food preparation ranges from partial prep, such as opening difficult jars, to cooking an entire meal. Similarly, gifts of food ranges from dropping off a few muffins to presenting a full course dinner. Home delivered meals refers to the federal program for homebound elders. Group meals includes both the federal congregate meal program and other regularly scheduled meal programs, such as soup kitchens. Eating at another person's home refers to invitations on a regular basis, once a month or more.

As Figure 10 demonstrates, the women in this study with greater functional limitations receive more help with food preparation, more likely receive home delivered meals, receive more gifts of food, and more typically eat at the homes of friends and relatives than women with few functional limitations. Attending group meals appears unrelated to functional status.

## Providers of Food and Meal Procurement Support

The major providers of food acquisition and meal preparation support are similar to the providers of diet support. An exception is the inclusion of homemaker aides, and the exclusion of physicians. Figure 11 shows the relationships of the helpers to the respondents. Friends and children account for almost $3/4$ of all helpers.

Figure 11: Relationship of food and meal procurement support providers (n=188) to respondents (n=88)

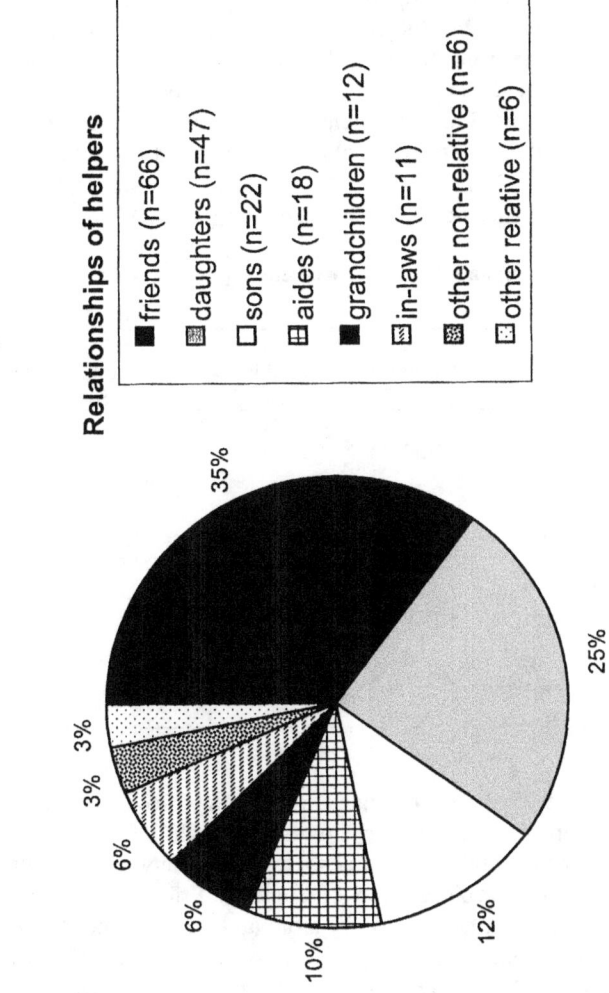

Subjects with BADL and IADL disabilities are more likely to receive food and meal procurement support than subjects with AADL or no disabilities ($\chi^2$=14.71, p=.001, $df$=1). Table 24 shows the number and percent of persons in each functional status category that receive food and meal procurement support.

The number of support providers and their relationships are also shown in Table 24. Subjects with BADL disabilities are most likely to receive help from home health aides. Otherwise, the relationship of support providers does not vary between functional status groups. The number of providers/recipient appears slightly larger for individuals with BADL and IADL disabilities than for those with AADL or no disabilities. However, the differences are not statistically significant (analysis of variance for unbalanced design [PROC GLM] p=.18).

**Table 24: Food and meal procurement support recipients and providers by functional status**

| Support | No Disabilities (n=13) | AADL Disabilities (n=27) | IADL Disabilities (n=29) | BADL Disabilities (n=33) |
|---|---|---|---|---|
| Recipients | 7 | 21 | 28 | 32 |
| % of n | 54 | 78 | 97 | 97 |
| Providers | | | | |
| Friends | 7 | 11 | 24 | 24 |
| Daughters | 5 | 14 | 12 | 16 |
| Sons | 0 | 4 | 11 | 7 |
| Aides | 0 | 0 | 3 | 15 |
| Other | 1 | 5 | 15 | 14 |
| Total | 13 | 34 | 65 | 76 |
| Total Providers/ Recipient | 1.9 | 1.6 | 2.3 | 2.4 |

Table 25 shows the specifics of which providers supply each type of instrumental support. Friends supply slightly fewer types of help per provider than children or aides. However many friends help, thus they are a considerable source of support. Friends are most noted for accompaniment to the grocery store and gifts of food. More than twice as many daughters help as sons, yet both offspring provide proportionally the same types of support. The respondents noted that their children are more likely than friends to invite them to dinner regularly and provide grocery shopping. Homemaker aides provide the most support per provider. They furnish the majority of in-home meal preparation.

**Table 25: Food and meal procurement support providers and types of support**

| Type of Support | Friends (n=66) | Daughters (n=47) | Sons (n=22) | Homemaker Aides (n=18) |
|---|---|---|---|---|
| Major grocery shopping | 6 | 7 | 6 | 5 |
| Grocery pick-ups | 18 | 16 | 7 | 9 |
| Accompaniment | 16 | 9 | 2 | 5 |
| Transportation | 25 | 18 | 6 | 6 |
| Food preparation | 3 | 1 | 2 | 9 |
| Food gifts | 25 | 10 | 3 | 1 |
| Meal invitations | 9 | 24 | 11 | 0 |
| Total | 102 | 85 | 37 | 35 |
| Types/Provider | 1.5 | 1.8 | 1.7 | 1.9 |

Table 25 includes 83% of the food and meal procurement support perceived by the respondents. The remaining 17% of the help is received from another 35 individuals representing four relationship categories: grandchildren, in-laws, other relative, and other nonrelative (see Figure 11).

Relatives other than children are not as likely to help. In this study only 29 other relatives, including brothers, sisters, cousins, grandchildren, and in-laws, provided instrumental support in comparison to the 69 children who provided support. However, when other relatives do help, they provide the same types and almost the same level of support, at 1.6 types/provider. Other relatives are less likely to extend meal invitations. Other nonrelatives only provided grocery delivery to the subjects, at 1.0 types/provider.

*Service Programs*

In addition to receiving help from individuals, the subjects in this study also report receiving help from programs. Only thirteen respondents use senior bus or public bus service for transportation to the grocery store, although over 75% do not drive. Many of the women expressed dissatisfaction with the bus systems. Some of the common issues include:

- shopping time limitation is too brief (usually 1 hour),
- the bus schedule conflicts with other events (such as congregate meal),
- concern over awkward/hazardous entry and exit from the bus,
- worry about acceptance by the clique that already rides the bus.

Meal program participation is shown in Table 26. Thirty-six percent of the women participate in meal programs. Generally, those who receive home delivered meals consider the program primarily a source of nutrition support. The participants in the congregate meal programs spoke of the social and financial benefits, in addition to the convenience of eating a healthful meal without the fuss of cooking.

**Table 26: Meal program participation**

| Type of Meal Program | No. Participating |
| --- | --- |
| Congregate meal program in housing complex | 8 |
| Congregate meal program off-site | 19 |
| Other meal program [a] | 5 |
| Home delivered meal program | 9 |
| None | 65 |
| Total [b] | 106 |

[a] Includes 1 @ soup kitchen, 3 @ local high school home economics lunch program, and 1 @ foster grandparent program.
[b] Four individuals participate in both home delivered meals and other meal programs. Therefore, total is greater than the number of subjects in this study.

Focus group subjects were asked about their perceptions of in-house lunch programs and off-site Senior Center lunches. The women stated that the menu was the biggest factor determining attendance. Food preferences, special diet needs, and food intolerances enter into their evaluation of the menu. Entertainment is a second determinant of attendance.

> "Once a week, on a Friday, we eat lunch there because after the meal they play BINGO and we love BINGO."

Others noted that activities at the location, such as a craft or a presentation, entice them to attend the meal.

Women who rarely or never participate in the lunches, stated that they prefer their own cooking and a more flexible schedule.

> "I don't like to know that at 11:45 every day I'm going to eat lunch, because sometimes I feel like it and sometimes I'm not here."

These women do not want to commit to the imposed schedule of the congregate meal. Some of the more impaired women indicated that they are never sure if they will feel energetic enough to attend on any given day.

Both participants and nonparticipants acknowledged social ramifications of meal program attendance.

> "We have cliques, which is not good. In other words, if you don't go, nobody else goes."

In addition to concerns about fitting in with the social strata at the lunches, there is worry over what others think. One focus group member declared that individuals who attend the lunch program *"are just damn good and lazy"* for not taking the trouble to prepare their own meals. The women do not wish to be the fodder for resident gossip.

Overall, the older women agreed that the congregate meals program is valuable. They felt that physically infirm adults and individuals that do not have the knowledge or interest in cooking healthful meals benefit the most from the program. The women stated that the price is reasonable and that the portion sizes are more than adequate.

## Satisfaction with Food and Meal Procurement Support

Only subjects who receive grocery acquisition support or meal preparation support are included in the analyses for satisfaction. Due to a misunderstanding by one of the interviewers, many women who do not receive help and a few who do receive help were excluded from questionnaire items regarding satisfaction with meal acquisition support. Thus, the analyses for satisfaction with food and meal procurement support are limited to individuals already involved in a task-specific support system. Because exploring satisfaction was one of the objectives of this study, the results are being reported. However, they should be interpreted with caution.

Most respondents who already receive help state that they are satisfied with the food and meal procurement support they receive. Only 12 of 77 individuals receiving grocery shopping help indicated that they would prefer more help in obtaining food. Only six of 45 women receiving meal preparation help would like more help in obtaining meals.

The associations between wanting more food and meal procurement support and demographic, health, and social variables were examined through correlation analyses. The specific variables included age, education, rent, self-rated health, number of years lived alone, number of years in present complex, functional status, BMI, social anchorage, total number of individuals who provide general support, and total number of individuals for whom subject provides support.

The only variable related to wanting more grocery shopping help was social anchorage (Spearman $r=-.33$, $p=.004$). That is, subjects who feel less socially embedded would like more help. A higher BMI was related to wanting more meal acquisition support (Spearman $r=.36$, $p=.007$). The average BMI for women who want more help is 32.7 in comparison to 27.7 for women who are satisfied with their current level of help.

Table 27 shows comparisons regarding the current level of help and satisfaction. No obvious differences are apparent between those who desire more support and those who are satisfied with the present level of support in the number of support providers, the relationships of the support providers, or the types of help received.

**Table 27: Women currently receiving food acquisition support — comparison between those who are satisfied and those who would prefer more support**

|  | Grocery Acquisition | | Meal Acquisition | |
|---|---|---|---|---|
|  | Want more (n=12) | Satisfied (n=65) | Want more (n=6) | Satisfied (n=39) |
| Number of Helpers |  |  |  |  |
| 1 | 4 | 34 | 4 | 23 |
| 2 | 6 | 22 | 0 | 11 |
| 3 | 0 | 4 | 1 | 4 |
| 4 | 2 | 3 | 1 | 0 |
| 5 | 0 | 2 | 0 | 1 |
| Primary Providers [a] |  |  |  |  |
| Friends | 5 | 35 | 2 | 26 |
| Daughters | 6 | 27 | 2 | 14 |
| Sons | 2 | 13 | 1 | 8 |
| Homemaker Aides | 2 | 14 | 3 | 6 |
| Types of Help [b] |  |  |  |  |
| Major Food Shopping | 3 | 11 |  |  |
| Grocery Pick-ups | 3 | 34 |  |  |
| Transportation | 6 | 25 |  |  |
| Accompaniment | 4 | 15 |  |  |
| Food Preparation |  |  | 1 | 5 |
| Food Gifts |  |  | 2 | 22 |
| Meal Invitations |  |  | 2 | 16 |
| Meal Program |  |  | 3 | 20 |

NOTE: Sample size is reduced because of interviewer erroneous omission of questions. See text for further details.
[a] Many individuals receive help from more than one source. Thus total of columns may be greater than total n.
[b] Many individuals receive more than one type of help, thus total of columns may be greater than total n.

## Discussion

Almost 90% of the participants in this study receive support in acquiring food or meals, either from individuals or from programs. The level of support varies with the needs of the elder. Women with more functional limitations generally receive greater amounts of aid than women with less functional impairment. Stoller and Pugliesi (1989) reported similar results from their longitudinal study of 85 informal support providers. The number of hours of general help and the number of tasks provided were associated with the functional status of the recipient. The researchers concluded that informal help providers are responsive to increasing needs of elders.

Of particular concern are two distinct groups of women involved in this study.

1. Women with low functional capabilities and meager sources of support. Are they able to obtain the food they need? What happens if their limited source of support fails?
2. Women with high functional capabilities, but absolutely no current food or meal acquisition support. In a difficult situation, would they request assistance? Would they "go without?" Or would they take a risky trip to the store?

Support from homemaker aides was notable for women with severe to moderate functional limitations. Otherwise, nearly all of the help from individuals was from informal sources, principally children and friends. Children are more likely to grocery shop for their mother and invite her to dinner on a regular basis. Friends bring gifts of food more often and provide accompaniment to the store.

Similar results were reported for a group of functionally disabled older adults who received home health services in Canada (Payette et al. 1995). In this group of 145 subjects, 94 older adults never did food shopping and 27 never prepared their own meals. Family and friends provided most of the help with grocery and meal acquisition. Only 12% of the Canadian sample received these services from formal sources.

The considerable and unique support which friends provide during the later years is currently gaining greater recognition (Antonucci and Akiyama 1995). The respondents in the present study perceive substantial support from their friends, most of whom live within the same apartment complex. The proximity and similar life situations may lead to frequent opportunities for supportive interactions.

The women in the present study also use formal nutrition support services. Participation in meal programs is higher than use of the senior bus service for grocery shopping. A frequent complaint regarding either service is the necessity to conform to a prearranged schedule.

Focus group subjects stated that they decide whether to attend senior lunch programs based on the menu, simultaneous activities, and social ramifications. Neyman, Zidenberg-Cherr, and McDonald (1996) reported that older adults in their study participated in congregate meal programs primarily for the opportunity to socialize. The second reason of the subjects was *"to eat a meal."* Yet, Walker and Beauchene (1991) found no relationship between loneliness scores of older adults and participation in group meal programs.

In contrast, individuals who receive home delivered meals are more impaired than congregate program subjects. These homebound recipients use Meals-on-Wheels primarily to meet their needs for nourishment (Biegel, Farkas, and Wadsworth 1994). Still, some food wastage occurs, mainly due to disliked taste (Fogler-Levitt et al. 1995). All of the respondents in this study who receive home delivered meals have moderate to severely impaired functional capabilities.

## COMPARISON WITH SUPPORT MODELS

Table 28 shows a summary of the nutrition support perceived by the women in this study. More than twice as many subjects receive support for food and meal procurement in comparison to support for modified diets. The respondents were able to recognize and discuss the instrumental types of support more easily than the emotional and informational types. Overall, 97 of the 102 women report help in obtaining food or help in following their diet.[1]

Suitor and Pillemer (1993) reported similar findings. They collected information on the types and providers of support to 95 female caregivers of elderly parents with dementia. Ninety-seven percent of the caregivers reported the receipt of instrumental types of help, while only 30% reported receipt of emotional support. The stressor and subsequent types of enacted support differ between our study and that of Suitor and Pillemer (1993). However, the ratio of instrumental to emotional help is quite close.

**Table 28: Summary of nutrition-related support by source**

|                  | Emotional/ Informational | Instrumental | | Combined |
|------------------|:---:|:---:|:---:|:---:|
|                  | Diet | Grocery | Meal | All |
| Receive Help     |      |         |      |     |
| Informal Only    | 20   | 58      | 29   | 38  |
| Formal Only      | 10   | 13      | 17   | 9   |
| Both             | 10   | 16      | 25   | 50  |
| Total            | 40   | 87      | 71   | 97  |
| Not Receive Help | 62   | 15      | 31   | 5   |

Most of the support to the elderly women in this study is received from informal sources. Forty-six percent of the women receive help from their friends, 41% receive help from their daughters, and 24% receive help from their sons. Fewer women report help from formal sources. Thirty-six percent participate in meal programs, 17% receive help from homemaker aides, and 13% receive support from their physicians. Daughters provide the most types of help per provider. However, the types of help they offer are distinct from the types of help from friends. For instance, daughters are the primary sources of advice, encouragement and meal invitations. Friends are the primary sources of self-disclosure and gifts of food.

A hierarchy of support providers and role specialization are common findings in investigations of social support (Dakof and Taylor 1990; Hogan and Eggebeen 1995; Troll 1994; Wellman and Wortley 1989). The two leading theories are a hierarchical-compensatory model and a task-specific model (Crohan and Antonucci 1989; Rook and Schuster 1996; Travis 1995). The hierarchical-compensatory model suggests that support providers are chosen on the basis of role relationships. Older adults prefer kin, followed by friends and neighbors, and lastly formal sources. In contrast, the task-specific model proposes that the nature of the task is most important. The preferred support provider is determined based on her ability to perform the needed function. In brief—instrumental, long-term support needs are provided by kin; crisis help and companionship are provided by friends; and technical skills are provided by formal sources.

Research results have upheld both models to a limited extent, but neither model fully (Rook and Schuster 1996). Studies have shown that informal sources provide 60 to 85% of the help (Chappell and Guse 1989; Kavesh 1986). The informal network is comprised of approximately 50% kin and 50% friends (Antonucci and Akiyama 1995; Armstrong and Goldsteen 1990). Most often, older adults report one leading support provider who also organizes other providers of support. The hierarchy of support providers descends from spouse to children, followed by friends, then siblings, then other relatives (Rook and Schuster 1996). Role specification is also noted. Antonucci and Akiyama (1995) propose that the obligatory nature of kin relations versus the optional nature of friend relations leads to task differentials.

The informal network is often viewed as the gateway to formal help, linking the elder to needed services (Chappell and Guse 1989). However, Noelker and Bass (1989) report that informal network members are as likely to avoid interactions with formal services. Formal support does appear to be the least utilized category of support (Chappell and Guse 1989). Typically, formal support begins to supplement informal support as the functional status of the elder declines (Hellman and Stewart 1994; Kelman, Thomas, and Tanaka 1994). However, characteristics of the support provider as well as characteristics of the elder influence service utilization (Noelker and Bass 1989).

The results of this study are consistent with the literature. Task specificity is evident, as well as a hierarchy of support providers. The majority of the support arises from informal sources, with family and friends about evenly divided. Disabled subjects are more likely to receive instrumental help from formal sources, such as home health aides and home delivered meals.

This study was cross sectional. The investigation of support patterns over time requires longitudinal data. Nonetheless, the differences across functional status categories in this sample of women suggest that nutrition-related support is responsive to changing needs in later life. The influence of the providers and types of nutrition-related support on actual diet quality is examined in the following chapters.

## NOTE

1. The group of five women who receive no help do not differ from the larger number of women who receive help on demographic, diet, or social variables, including functional status, age, years lived alone, education, rent, years at complex, BMI, number of diet modifications, origin of diet, overall help received, reciprocal help, and social anchorage. In other words, this small group appears to have the same need for nutrition support, are not socially isolated, yet receive no nutrition help.

Comparisons were also examined between the nine women who receive help from formal sources only and the remaining 88 who receive help from informal or combined sources. Again, no differences exist on any of the aforementioned variables, except functional status. As a group, the women who receive formal help only are higher functioning. Most of these women are involved in congregate meals or use Senior Van service.

CHAPTER 6
# Food Intake and Dietary Adequacy

The analytic research goal of this dissertation was to investigate the relationship between nutrition-related social support and diet quality. Attributes of nutrition-related social support were described in detail in the previous chapters. In this chapter, attributes of respondent diets are discussed.

The primary intent was to examine how social support might influence overall food intake patterns. Food intake determines nutritional quality of the diet, and hence nutritional status of the individual. Thus, usual food patterns were assessed using a food frequency instrument. Typical food intake is described below, as well as average nutrient intake from foods. Because of the focus on foodways, contributions from vitamin/mineral supplements were not examined. As in previous chapters, comparisons with similar research samples and national groups are discussed. Implications of the current eating patterns are explored. Summary diet quality measures are defined and described.

## FOOD PATTERNS

The subjects in this study completed a modified version of the NCI food frequency questionnaire (Block et al. 1986). Use of this instrument permits examination of typical food patterns as well as nutrient intakes. Figure 12 shows the 10 foods eaten most frequently by this group. Bread is the most commonly consumed item, with an average intake of 12 servings per week. Most of the respondents habitually eat breakfast. Many foods commonly eaten at the first meal of the day appear in the top 10 list (toast, coffee, tea, cold cereal, milk and orange juice).

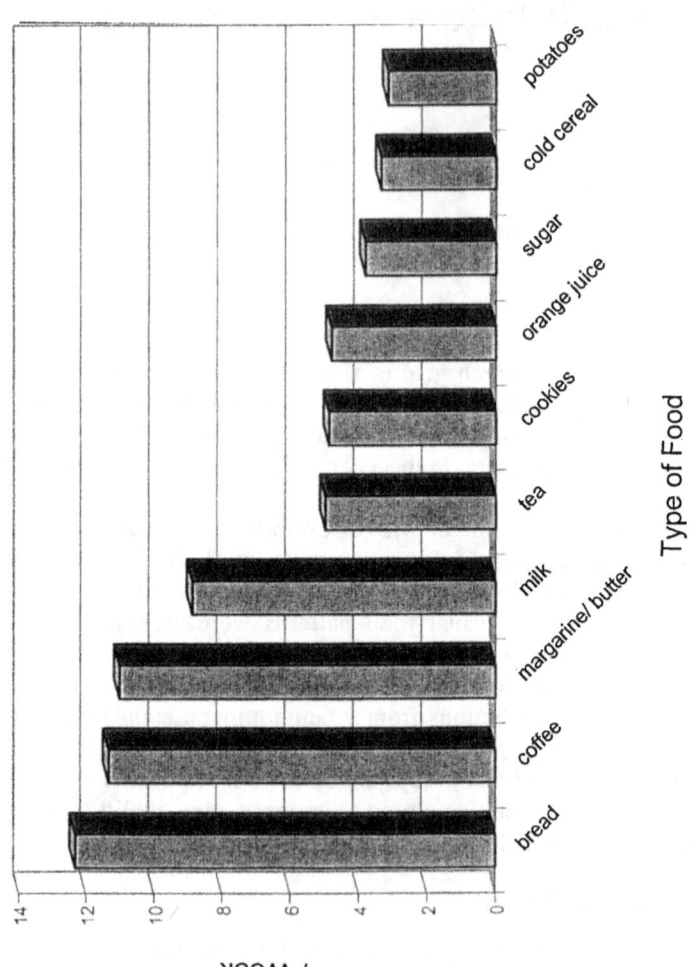

Figure 12: Average consumption per week of the ten most frequently eaten foods

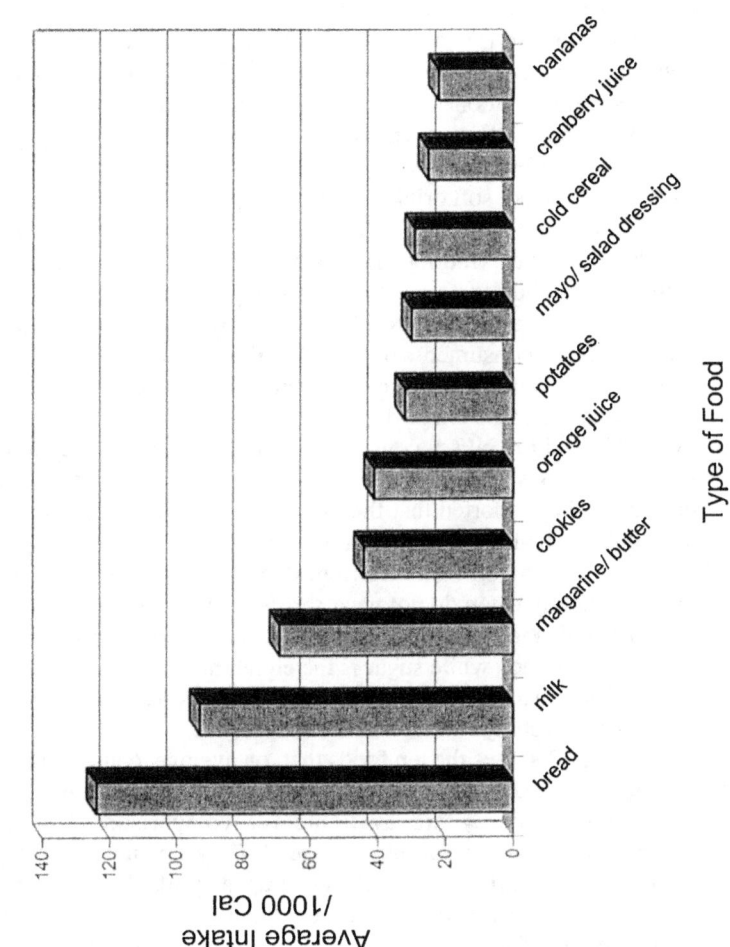

Figure 13: Average intake per 1000 calories of the ten highest contributing foods

Interestingly, these core foods appear quite similar to those of elderly women 20 years ago. Fanelli and Stevenhagen (1985) categorized the food items reported in three-day food records by participants in the 1977–78 National Food Consumption Survey (NFCS). The top ten core foods of females over 75 years in descending order were bread, milk, ground coffee, margarine, sugar, instant coffee, tea, potatoes, orange juice, and eggs.

In comparison, Block et al. (1985) reported the most frequently consumed foods from the NHANES II (1976–80). These results were obtained from a nationally representative sample of individuals age 19–74 years. The foods most frequently consumed by the whole group in descending order were coffee/tea, bread, margarine, milk, cookies, sugar, green salad, soft drinks, cheeses, and eggs.

Some variation in the order of the food items between Fanelli's, Block's, and our findings is attributable to minor food grouping differences. Thus the core food lists appear to be more alike than different, especially in the top five items. However, the individuals in the NHANES consumed salads, soft drinks, and cheese much more frequently. Whether these differences are due to participant characteristics or the era of data collection is uncertain. The subjects of this study and the NFCS consumed orange juice more frequently than the NHANES sample. Many of the subjects in this study are on diuretics. They reported that they needed to consume sufficient orange juice daily to maintain potassium balance.

Both serving size and nutrient density vary by food. The foods most frequently eaten do not necessarily have a proportional impact on the quality of the diet. For instance, the usual serving size of sugar is very small. In fact, while sugar is the eighth most commonly consumed food, it only accounts for 0.5% of the average caloric intake of the women in this study.

Figure 13 shows the ten foods that, on average, contribute the most calories to the diets of study participants. Only the results from the NHANES II survey are available for comparison. The top ten contributors of energy for persons age 19–74 years in descending order were bread, cookies, alcoholic beverages, milk, hamburgers, beef steaks/roasts, soft drinks, hot dogs/ham, eggs, and french fries. Considerable differences are noted between the consumption pattern of the NHANES group and this study sample. The distinctions are again likely attributable to both differences in participant characteristics and in the era of data collection.

In general, the respondents in this study appear to have implemented some current dietary recommendations. The women drink more skim and 1% milk than 2% or whole milk. Their intake of soft margarine exceeds that of stick margarine. They eat poultry in preference to beef or pork. On average, this group consumes less than two eggs per week.

However, some areas for improvement are apparent. These subjects eat over twice as much white bread as whole grain bread. They consume more servings of cookies than servings of apples, pears, oranges, and bananas combined. They have a high intake of empty calorie foods, such as jello, soda, and fruit flavored drinks. On average, these women eat cooked greens only once per month. The nutrient intakes reflect these food patterns.

## NUTRIENT INTAKES

The mean energy intake of these respondents is 1296 calories/day, ranging from 557 to 2567 calories. Mean caloric intake in relation to body weight is 20 calories/kg/day, ranging from 7 to 42 calories/kg. Similar calorie intakes have been found in other groups of elderly women, as assessed by food frequency questionnaires (Holcomb 1995; Mares-Perlman et al. 1993; Patterson, Haines, and Popkin 1996) and diet records (Coulston, Craig, and Voss 1996; Walker and Beauchene 1991).

In general, the macronutrient and micronutrient intakes of the subjects in this study are consistent with findings from previous studies of elderly women. In Table 29 the intakes of these subjects are compared with the intakes of a nationally representative group of elderly women who completed the 1987 National Health Interview Survey (NHIS) (Block and Subar 1992). The NHIS included a 60–item version of the NCI food frequency questionnaire. NHIS results are adjusted to compensate for use of the short interview form.

**Table 29: Mean ±SE nutrient intakes of subjects in comparison to adjusted intakes of a nationally representative sample (Block and Subar 1992)**

| Nutrient | Subject Intakes | National Sample | |
|---|---|---|---|
| | Women 75–95 (n=102) | Women 65–79 (n=1926) | Women 80+ (n=521) |
| Calories (kcal) | 1296±41.3 | 1295±11.5 | 1308±17.0 |
| Fat (g) | 48.1±2.3 | 50.7±0.6 | 50.5±0.8 |
| Protein (g) | 47.3±1.5 | 51.3±0.6 | 50.4±0.8 |
| Carbohydrate (g) | 171.9±5.6 | 156.6±1.5 | 163±2.5 |
| Fiber (g) | 10.6±0.38 | 10.5±0.12 | 10.3±0.18 |
| Vitamins | | | |
| Vitamin A (IU) | 5525±216 | 5572±79 | 5476±153 |
| Vitamin E (mg) | 6.5±0.34 | 5.2±0.06 | 5.2±0.13 |
| Vitamin C (mg) | 129±8.5 | 105±1.8 | 104±2.8 |
| Thiamin (mg) | 1.0±0.03 | 1.0±0.01 | 1.0±0.02 |
| Riboflavin (mg) | 1.4±0.05 | 1.4±0.02 | 1.4±0.03 |
| Niacin (mg) | 12.8±0.38 | 14.5±0.16 | 14.2±0.23 |
| Vitamin B6 (mg) | 1.2±0.04 | N/A [a] | N/A |
| Folacin (µg) | 225±9.2 | 205±2.1 | 205±4.1 |
| Minerals | | | |
| Calcium (mg) | 677±33 | 617±10 | 621±14 |
| Iron (mg) | 9.2±0.34 | 10.3±0.10 | 10.3±0.17 |
| Magnesium (mg) | 232.4±7.02 | N/A | N/A |
| Phosphorus (mg) | 882±32 | 886±11 | 873±15 |
| Sodium (mg) | 2252±83 | 1984±22 | 2034±31 |
| Zinc (mg) | 6.4±0.24 | N/A | N/A |

[a] N/A Intake not reported in reference article.

Most of the mean nutrient intake levels are similar between these subjects and the NHIS nationally representative sample. On average, the respondents in this study report consuming slightly less protein, niacin, and iron than the national group. However, the intakes of vitamins E and C, folate, calcium, and sodium appear slightly higher in this sample than in the NHIS participants. Overall, the differences are slight.

To determine the adequacy of the diet, nutrient intakes of the study subjects are compared to existing standards:

- 1989 Recommended Dietary Allowances (RDA)(FNB 1989)
- Dietary Guidelines for Americans (USDA 1995).

The RDAs are recommended nutrient intake levels determined to meet the needs of practically all healthy persons in the U.S. They can be used to evaluate if the group of elderly study subjects is at risk for a deficient intake of vitamins and minerals. The Dietary Guidelines for Americans address the problems associated with over consumption. The Guidelines set forth dietary recommendations to promote health and aid in the prevention of prevalent chronic diseases.

## Comparison to RDAs

Table 30 presents the calorie and nutrient intakes of these respondents in comparison to the 1989 RDAs. Nutrient intake of the subjects only reflects nutrients from foods; the use of vitamin and mineral supplements was not assessed.

No absolute RDA value is proposed for caloric intake in individuals over 75 years of age. Regardless, adequacy of dietary calories is best determined by examining energy balance. Only three of the study subjects reported unexplained, persistent weight loss during the past five years. The majority complained of "unexplained" weight gain. As discussed in Chapter 3, many more of these women are overweight than underweight.

### Protein

The 1989 RDA for protein is based on 0.8 g/kg body weight. However, recent research findings, including nitrogen balance studies and functional outcome measures, suggest that 1.0 g/kg body weight may be more desirable for the older age group (Bidlack and Wang 1995; Campbell and Evans 1996; Campbell et al. 1994; McBride 1995). The increase in the protein requirement may reflect decreased dietary protein utilization combined with elevated needs due to emotional stress and physical illness. Furthermore, visceral organs, which experience increased protein turnover in comparison to muscle, account for a greater percentage of lean body mass in the elderly (Schlenker 1998).

**Table 30: Nutrient intakes in comparison to 1989 RDAs (FNB 1989)**

| Nutrient | RDA [a] | Subject Intakes | | |
|---|---|---|---|---|
| | | Mean ± SD | Range | % consuming < 2/3 RDA |
| Calories (kcal) | N/A [b] | 1296±417 | (557–2567) | — |
| Protein (g) | 50 | 47.3±15.2 | (22.1–97.5) | 19 |
| Vitamins | | | | |
| Vitamin A (µg RE) | 800 | 852.1±277.3 | (180.3–1676.5) | 9 |
| Vitamin E (mg) | 8 | 6.5±3.4 | (2.6–26.6) | 45 |
| Vitamin C (mg) | 60 | 128.8±85.5 | (15.7–673.1) | 6 |
| Thiamin (mg) | 1.0 | 1.0±0.3 | (0.4–2.1) | 16 |
| Riboflavin (mg) | 1.2 | 1.4±0.5 | (0.6–3.2) | 7 |
| Niacin (mg) | 13 | 12.8±3.8 | (5.3–27.9) | 12 |
| Vitamin B6 (mg) | 1.6 | 1.2±0.4 | (0.4–2.4) | 45 |
| Folate (µg) | 180 | 224.6±92.7 | (72.6–661.7) | 4 |
| Minerals | | | | |
| Calcium (mg) | 800 | 677.3±329.5 | (209.4–1951.0) | 34 |
| Iron (mg) | 10 | 9.2±3.4 | (3.5–24.8) | 21 |
| Magnesium (mg) | 280 | 232.4±70.9 | (90.3–452.7) | 29 |
| Phosphorus (mg) | 800 | 882.0±327.1 | (334.5–2132.3) | 10 |
| Zinc (mg) | 12 | 6.4±2.5 | (2.7–19.3) | 80 |

[a] Recommended dietary allowances for healthy females age 51+. The Food and Nutrition Board that establishes the RDAs concluded that present data is inadequate to formulate separate recommendations for an older age group.
[b] Recommended calorie level for females 51–75 years is 1900 calories. Women over 75 years are expected to require less energy intake due to reduced lean body mass and reduced activity. However, no specific level was established.

The average intake for this group of women is 0.7 g/kg/day, ranging from 0.3 to 1.3g/kg. The calculated levels of protein indicate that intake of this nutrient may be suboptimal for many of the participants. Campbell et al. (1994) suggests that chronic, marginally low levels of protein intake may compromise immunocompetence and contribute to the loss in lean body mass associated with aging. Thus, the low protein intake of many of these subjects could result in delayed healing from surgery or infection. Of equal importance is the potential loss of muscle mass and eventual loss of muscle function necessary to accomplish the tasks of daily living (McBride 1995).

# Food Intake and Dietary Adequacy

## *Nutrients*

The nutrients that appear the least adequate in this group of women include vitamins E and B6 and the minerals calcium, magnesium and zinc. Low intakes of these nutrients are fairly typical in older adults. Large surveys have documented intakes below 2/3 RDA in 40–60% of elderly individuals (Bidlack and Wang 1995). Although low intakes may be typical, they are nonetheless undesirable.

## Zinc

Zinc intake appears the most inadequate. The mean intake is only half the RDA and the vast majority of respondents are consuming less than 2/3 the recommended amount of this mineral. In general, zinc directly correlates with calorie and especially protein intakes (Bidlack and Wang 1995). The low zinc intake of these subjects is therefore anticipated in light of their low energy and protein consumption.

The few researchers who have reported zinc intake in older adults have noted similar low levels (Mares-Perlman et al. 1993; Neyman, Zidenberg-Cherr, and McDonald 1996; Nieman et al. 1989). Neyman, Zidenberg-Cherr, and McDonald (1996) also documented low serum zinc concentrations in almost one quarter of their elderly sample. Zinc deficiency is traditionally associated with diminished taste acuity, delayed wound healing and impaired immunity (Schlenker 1998). The functional significance of marginally low intakes of zinc is currently unknown (Ahmed 1992).

## Vitamin B6

The dietary intake of vitamin B6 is also frequently found to be low in studies of the elderly (Ahmed 1992; Bidlack and Wang 1995). In younger individuals, vitamin B6 requirements vary with the level of protein intake. However, the B6 needs of older individuals may be independent of protein consumption (Schlenker 1998). Vitamin B6 is essential for the metabolism of proteins (including homocysteine), optimal immune function (including lymphocyte and interleukin-2 production), and maximal cognitive functioning (including abstract reasoning) (La Rue et al. 1997; Russell 1997). Previous researchers have noted that low-income is associated with poorer vitamin B6 intake

(Russell and Suter 1993). In agreement, a significant number of women in this low-income sample appear to be consuming inadequate levels of vitamin B6.

Vitamin E

Vitamin E intake was also poor in this group of participants. Similarly, the mean intake of 6.31 mg in older women in the 1988–91 NHANES III (Schlenker 1998) and the mean intake of 5.2 mg in older females in the NHIS (Block and Subar 1992) were below the RDA. However, researchers have not found low plasma tocopherol levels in elderly women (Ahmed 1992; Bidlack and Wang 1995; Russell and Suter 1993).

Vitamin E is a potent antioxidant, preventing the degradation of unsaturated fatty acids by free radicals (FNB 1989). Thus, the requirement for vitamin E varies with the level of polyunsaturated fatty acid (PUFA) in the diet. Currently the RDA is based on a ratio of 0.4 mg tocopherol/g PUFA. The subjects in this study did meet the ratio recommendation, at approximately 0.42 mg tocopherol/g PUFA. However, Murphy, Subar, and Block (1990) caution that a fixed ratio may be misleading. The ratio between vitamin E and PUFA is not linear at extremes of intake. Furthermore, the number of unsaturated double bonds may influence tocopherol needs (FNB 1989).

Calcium

Many food intake studies of the elderly have analyzed for the calcium content of the diet. Almost all have reported low intakes of calcium in relation to the RDA. Table 31 shows a sample of the values reported for various groups of older adults. Generally, the average calcium intake runs between 600 to 700 mg, while the 1989 RDA stands at 800 mg. As reported in Table 31, only the healthy, highly educated group of women interviewed by Zipp and Holcomb (1992) had a mean intake above the RDA. However, these researchers noted that even in this health conscious group, the intakes of half the women were below the recommended value of 800 mg.

**Table 31: Calcium intakes—comparison with other groups of elderly women**

| Research Group | Sample Characteristics | Food Intake Method [a] | Calcium Mean ± SE |
|---|---|---|---|
| This study | n=102, age 75–95, low-income | FFQ | 677±33 |
| Block-1992 | n=1926, age 65–79, natl. sample | FFQ | 617±10 |
|  | n=521, age 80+, national sample | FFQ | 621±14 |
| Mares-Perlman-1993 | n=211, age 65–84, random sample | FFQ | 584±290 (SD [b]) |
| Neyman-1996 | n=47, age 60–89, congregate meal participants | 3D | 622±38 |
|  | n=44, age 60–89, nonparticipants | 3D | 718±44 |
| Nieman-1989 | n=23, age 65–80, vegetarians | 7D | 626±40 |
|  | n=14, age 65–80, nonvegetarians | 7D | 633±73 |
| Posner-1987 | n=35, age 63–99, homebound | 24h | 510±396 (SD) |
| Walker-1991 | n=61, age 60–94, independent | 3D | 661±40 |
| Zipp-1992 | n=100, age 65+, healthy, active, highly educated | FFQ | 936±488 (SD) |

[a] FFQ = food frequency questionnaire
3D = 3–day food record
7D = 7–day food record
24h = 24 hour recall.
[b] SD rather than SE reported in reference article.

Approximately 99% of the calcium in the adult is found in the skeleton, the remainder is in the blood and tissues (FNB 1989). Serum calcium levels are tightly controlled to maintain vital nerve, muscle, and cellular functions. Several hormones, including parathyroid hormone, estrogen, testosterone, and calcitriol (vitamin D), regulate calcium absorption and secretion, as well as bone resorption and formation. During the later years, resorption predominates over formation. For women eating typical U.S. diets, bone loss averages approximately 3% per year the first few years following menopause (Dawson-Hughes 1997). Afterwards, the loss slows to about 1% per year.

A low intake of calcium has been associated with the bone loss of osteoporosis and subsequent fractures (Ahmed 1992). The recently proposed Dietary Reference Intakes of the FNB propose an Adequate Intake of 1200 mg/day for females 70+ years (Schlicker et al. 1997). The National Institute of Health Consensus Development Panel has recommended 1500 mg/day for postmenopausal women not taking estrogen and 1000 mg/day for postmenopausal women taking estrogen (Packard and Heaney 1997).

Magnesium

The mean intake of magnesium in this study was only 83% of the RDA. Almost one-third of the subjects consumed less than 67% RDA. Dietary intake studies, such as the NHANES III have shown decreasing intakes of magnesium with increasing age (Bidlack and Wang 1995; Schlenker 1998). However, blood levels appear relatively constant between younger and older subjects.

Magnesium is involved in the metabolism of energy, the transmission of nerve impulses, and the activation of enzymes (FNB 1989; Schlenker 1998). Researchers are also examining possible associations between magnesium and certain chronic diseases, such as diabetes mellitus, hypertension, and osteoporosis. Diabetes, chronic alcoholism, laxative abuse and certain diuretics increase magnesium excretion. These predisposing factors may be more prevalent in the elderly than in younger individuals.

Folate

Based on research findings specific to the elderly, Russell (1997) has suggested revisions to the RDAs for older adults. His recommendations are displayed in Table 32 (also discussed by Guigoz 1995). The proposed changes to the RDAs for riboflavin and vitamin A would not substantially alter the at-risk status for these subjects. The recommended increases to the B6 and calcium RDAs indicate that an even greater proportion of this sample has inadequate intakes than previously discussed. Similarly, the suggested increase to the folate RDA indicates that many of these respondents are consuming inadequate amounts.

**Table 32: Suggested revisions to the RDAs for elderly females (Russell 1997)—in comparison to intakes in this study**

| Nutrient | Current RDA | New Recommendation (Russell 1997) | This Study Mean ± SD |
|---|---|---|---|
| Riboflavin (mg) | 1.2 | "Same or higher" (1.3?) | 1.4±0.5 |
| Vitamin B6 (mg) | 1.6 | 1.9 | 1.2±0.4 |
| Folate (µg) | 180 | 400 | 224±92.7 |
| Calcium (mg) | 800 | "Considerably higher" (1500?) | 677±330 |
| Vitamin A (µg RE) | 800 | "Same or lower" | 852±277 |

By January 1998, the FDA mandated that all enriched white flour, pasta, cornmeal, grits, and white rice be fortified with folate (Koehler et al. 1997). The mandate was implemented to help women of childbearing years consume adequate folate to reduce the incidence of neural tube birth defects. The mandate may also help older adults consume increased levels of folate. Folate intake is inversely related to serum homocysteine concentration – and elevated levels of homocysteine are related to increased risk for cardiovascular disease. Thus, the subjects of this study would appear to benefit from folate fortification and other means of improved folate intake.

## Comparison to Dietary Guidelines

Comparison of nutrient intakes with the RDAs permits identification of deficiencies. The Dietary Guidelines for Americans address the problems of overconsumption. Table 33 shows how the diets of study subjects compare with the recommendations of the Dietary Guidelines.

**Table 33: Diet patterns in comparison to the Dietary Guidelines (U.S.DA 1995)**

|  | Guideline | Subject Intakes | | |
| --- | --- | --- | --- | --- |
|  |  | Mean ± SD | Range | % Not Meeting Guideline |
| Sodium (mg) | ≤ 2400 | 2252.2±842.5 | (608–4697) | 37 |
| Fat (%) | ≤ 30 % calories | 32.6±8.3 | (16.5–56.7) | 59 |
| Saturated fat (%) | ≤10 % calories | 10.5±3.8 | (4.4–25.2) | 44 |
| Cholesterol (mg) | ≤ 300 | 155.3±91.0 | (36–651) | 7 |
| Servings alcohol | ≤ 2 | 0.1±0.3 | (0.0–2.0) | 0 |
| Fiber (g) | 20 - 35 | 10.6±3.8 | (2.9–21.0) | 98 |

In these elderly women, an excess of calories from fat is notable. However, the 33% of calories from fat found in the diets of these women is preferable to the 34–37% in the usual American diet. Decreased sodium and saturated fat intakes could also benefit a substantial portion of the participants. In contrast, the low cholesterol and alcohol intakes of the group are commendable.

High fat diets, especially those high in saturated fat and cholesterol have been linked to a number of poor health outcomes, including:

- hypertension and thus cardiovascular disease (Kuller 1997);
- certain cancers, especially colon, breast and ovarian, prostate and pancreas (Harrison 1997; Kuller 1997);
- obesity, associated with non-insulin dependent diabetes, gout, gallbladder disease, and osteoarthritis, as well as cardiovascular disease and some cancers (Ernst et al. 1997; Ravussin and Tataranni 1997).

Diets high in sodium increase the risk of hypertension in salt-sensitive individuals. A meta-analysis by Cutler, Follmann, and Allender (1997), not only determined that salt-sensitivity is real, but furthermore indicated that most of the U.S. population is salt-sensitive to some degree. Ely (1997) has proposed stress as a mediator of salt-sensitivity. While the average salt intake of this group of respondents was within recommended levels, almost 40% might benefit from a decrease in consumption.

Dietary fiber is the remaining weak area in the diets of the respondents. In general, Americans do not consume enough fiber rich foods. These subjects are no exception. The mean intake is half the recommended level with only two respondents consuming suggested amounts. Adequate fiber intake is associated with a decreased incidence of cardiovascular disease, diabetes, and certain cancers (Schlenker 1998; Weisburger 1997). Fiber from all sources is important—including beans, grains, fruits, and vegetables.

## IMPLICATIONS

The levels of nutrient intake suggest that clinical deficiency disorders, such as scurvy or pellagra, would be uncommon in this group of elderly women. However, the patterns of nutrient intake, especially the insufficiencies and excesses noted above, are associated with undesirable health outcomes.

Currently, cardiovascular heart disease (CHD) is the leading cause of death in the United States. A diet rich in fat, especially saturated fat, and low in fiber and antioxidants (vitamins A, C, and E) is associated with increased morbidity and mortality due to CHD (Kwiterovich 1997). The diet of this group of elderly women matches the high risk profile. The dietary risk factors for cancer, the second leading cause of death, are similar with the addition of a high intake of cured meats. Again, the diet of the study subjects places them at high risk.

Of the antioxidants, vitamin E intake was the lowest in these respondents. In addition to decreasing susceptibility to cardiovascular disease and cancer, this vitamin is known to boost immunity to infectious diseases and cataracts. Through different processes, vitamin B6 and zinc also appear to boost immune function. For these elderly women, any reduction in morbidity can greatly increase the quality of their lives.

Bone fractures due to mineral loss are an aggravating condition suffered by many older women. The low calcium intake of this group is a known risk factor contributing to the incidence of osteoporosis. Adequate vitamin D is also essential to maintain bone mass. The functional limitations of the respondents coupled with the harsh winter climate in Eastern Connecticut would suggest that cutaneous vitamin D synthesis would be insufficient during much of the year. Of concern are the high medical costs, the loss of independence and the high risk of mortality that follow osteoporotic fractures.

The diet profile of this group of women places them at high risk for morbidity and mortality resulting from CHD, cancer, and osteoporosis. Furthermore, immune systems may be less efficient. Individually, the risk for these health outcomes varies with additional lifestyle and hereditary factors.

Other dietary problems are apparent for specific individuals. While these problems may not be common, they should not be overlooked. For example, Irene habitually avoids a wide variety of fruits and vegetables because of serious gastrointestinal problems. As a result, her average vitamin A intake is only 180 RE/day. This amount is far below the minimum felt necessary to maintain plasma levels (FNB 1989). A chronic intake at this low level would be expected to deplete liver stores, eventually resulting in vision abnormalities.

Hazel offers a second example. She suffers from hypertension. Years ago, her doctor recommended a low salt diet and prescribed Vasotec. However, her present sodium intake, including an estimate of table salt, averages 4590 mg/day. If Hazel is salt sensitive and she decreases her consumption of high salt foods, she could possibly reduce or even eliminate the Vasotec.

In summary, many of these respondents eat a diet that places them at risk for chronic degenerative disorders. Furthermore, analyses of individual diets show problem areas specific to the special needs of each person. Undesirable health consequences may result which could have been prevented through diet modification.

## DIETARY QUALITY

For this study, a summary measure of dietary quality was necessary to examine the relationship with social support. At this time, no single measure has been proposed that optimally conveys the complexity of the diet and its associations with biochemical, anthropometric, and health parameters (Kant 1996). In a recent review, Kant (1996) reported that most measures are based solely on the nutrient content of the diet;

a few are food or food-group based. Only three indices were found that combine nutrients and foods.

Two summary measures were selected for use in this study, the Mean Adequacy Ratio (MAR) and the Diet Quality Index (DQI). The MAR has been frequently employed in dietary studies as an index of overall nutrient adequacy. The score reflects the intake of 11 key nutrients in comparison to the Recommended Dietary Allowances (Gibson 1990). Figure 14 displays the details of the MAR calculations.

**Figure 14: Mean Adequacy Ratio (Gibson 1990)**

The Mean Adequacy Ratio is the average of the Nutrient Adequacy Ratios (NARs). **Nutrient Adequacy Ratios** are calculated as:

$$NAR = \frac{\text{Individual's daily intake of a nutrient}}{\text{RDA of that nutrient}}$$

The 11 nutrients used in these calculations include protein, vitamin A, thiamin, riboflavin, folacin, vitamin B6, vitamin C, calcium, magnesium, iron and zinc.

Any individual nutrient intakes in excess of 100% of the RDA are truncated at 1.0. The Mean Adequacy Ratio for each subject is then calculated as:

$$MAR = \frac{\text{Sum of the NARs for 11 nutrients}}{11}$$

The resultant summary score is indicative of overall nutrient adequacy of the diet.

In contrast, the DQI portrays nutrient and food group intake in comparison to the Dietary Guidelines (Patterson, Haines, and Popkin 1994). The scoring method was recently developed to provide an indicator of dietary risk for the chronic diseases. However, the method has been criticized for weighting fat intake too heavily (Kant 1996). Regardless, the DQI is one of very few methods that reflect both nutrient and nonnutrient constituents of the diet. Table 34 shows the details of the DQI.

**Table 34: Diet Quality Index (Patterson, Haines, and Popkin 1994)**

The Diet Quality Index is the sum of scores for each of the eight categories. The total DQI represents a dietary pattern score indicating nutritional risk of chronic diseases.

| Recommendation | | Score |
|---|---|---|
| Total fat | ≤ 30% total calories | 0 |
| | 30–40 % | 1 |
| | > 40% | 2 |
| Saturated fat | ≤ 10% total calories | 0 |
| | 10–13% | 1 |
| | >13% | 2 |
| Cholesterol | ≤300 mg | 0 |
| | 300–400 mg | 1 |
| | > 400 mg | 2 |
| Servings of fruits and vegetables | 5 + servings | 0 |
| | 3–4 | 1 |
| | 0–2 | 2 |
| Servings of grains and legumes | 6 + servings | 0 |
| | 4–5 | 1 |
| | 0–3 | 2 |
| Protein [a] | ≤ 100% RDA | 1 |
| | 100–150% | 0 |
| | > 150% | 2 |
| Sodium | ≤ 2,400 mg | 0 |
| | 2,400–3,400 mg | 1 |
| | > 3,400 mg | 2 |
| Calcium | ≥ 100% RDA | 0 |
| | 66–99% RDA | 1 |
| | < 65% RDA | 2 |

[a] The "1" and "0" scores for this study were reversed from the original scoring assignments of the DQI. Current recommendations for this elderly age group are to consume 1.0 g protein/kg body weight. Thus 100–150% RDA appears optimal for these study participants.

The mean MAR and DQI scores are shown in Table 35. Please note that higher MAR scores indicate better nutrient adequacy. DQI is the reverse. Lower DQI scores indicate a more healthful diet.

**Table 35: Dietary scores**

| Dietary Index | Mean ± SD | Range |
|---|---|---|
| MAR | 81.8 ± 12.7 | 50.3 - 100.0 |
| DQI | 6.4 ± 2.4 | 2.0 - 12.0 |

Several researchers have employed the MAR in analyses of their data, but none have reported the distribution of MAR scores in their samples (Guthrie and Scheer 1981; Krebs-Smith et al. 1987; Toner 1987; Walker and Beauchene 1991). Thus, no comparisons are available for the MAR summary statistics of Table 35.

Popkin, Siega-Riz, and Haines (1996) calculated DQI scores from the 24-hour diet recall data of several national surveys. They categorized participants by ethnicity and SES, but not by gender. The most analogous subgroup comparisons are displayed in Table 36. The mean of the participants in this study is similar to the mean of the 1989–91 national data. However, more women in this study have scores of 10 or greater, indicating a larger proportion with a poor diet than in the national samples.

**Table 36: Diet Quality Index scores—comparison with national data**

|  | Subjects | Mean ± SEE | Score ≤4 % | Score ≥10 % |
|---|---|---|---|---|
| This study | 102 F age 75–95 | 6.4 ± 0.24 | 22.5 | 11.8 |
| 1965 NFCS | 2146 M+F age 18+ | 7.2 ± 0.03 | 9.3 | 10.7 |
| 1977–78 NFCS | 3144 M+F age 18+ | 6.8 ± 0.03 | 12.9 | 6.7 |
| 1989–91 NHANES III | 3195 M+F age 18+ | 6.3 ± 0.03 | 19.9 | 4.4 |

NOTE: Comparison groups are low SES participants in three nationally representative surveys (Popkin, Siega-Riz, and Haines 1996)

Typically, dietary quality is related to socioeconomic indices and age. However, the recruitment procedures for this study were designed to control these influences. Accordingly, no significant associations were found between either summary score and the respondent's age, rent, or education (examined with Pearson's correlation coefficient or

Spearman's rho). Self-rated health, the number of years of living alone and the number of years in the present apartment complex were not associated with dietary quality either.

## DISCUSSION AND CONCLUSIONS

The interviewers and subjects in this study worked hard to obtain a true picture of the respondent's usual diet. The subjects enjoyed reporting their food patterns. They explained in detail their shopping habits, meals and recipes. Typically, the food frequency took over an hour to complete, more than twice the expected time for completion (Smucker et al. 1989).

The NCI food frequency questionnaire is acclaimed as both a reliable and valid indicator of food and nutrient intakes (Block et al. 1986; Block et al. 1990; Block et al. 1992; Cummings et al. 1987; Mares-Perlman et al. 1993). The degree to which it approximates the true diet has been likened to approximately 3 to 5 days of diet records (Block et al. 1990; Liu 1994). To further increase accuracy, several options were employed.

- Inclusion of population-based portion sizes as small, medium, or large (Block et al. 1992).
- Interviewer administered to improve recall and decrease reporting and coding errors (Smucker et al. 1989).
- Inclusion of an open-ended section to capture the complete diet (Zulkifli and Yu 1992).
- Adjustment and summary questions to provide clarifications of usual intake and checks on total consumption patterns (Block et al. 1986; Patterson, Haines, and Popkin 1996).

However, food intake records inevitably contain some error. For food frequencies, respondents are particularly prone to overestimating the intakes of foods commonly eaten as well as foods with a healthy connotation (Salvini et al. 1989; Zulkifli and Yu 1992). Respondents are more likely to underestimate the intakes of foods seldom eaten and foods that are considered unhealthy. In addition, vitamin/mineral supplements were not examined. Supplements would increase the levels of intake for some nutrients.

The dietary analysis therefore approximates the attributes of the true diet. The magnitude of identified problems could be slightly more or slightly less severe. Furthermore, dietary reference standards are unavailable. The RDAs are not specific for women in the age range of this study. In addition, the RDAs are intended as recommendations for healthy persons. Over 95% of these respondents reported one or more illnesses.

Because of the analytical limitations, interpretation of the diets of these women must proceed with caution. However, many of the problem areas identified here are supported by findings with other groups of elderly women using a variety of dietary intake methods. Typically, protein intakes are marginal; vitamin E, B6, calcium, magnesium and zinc are inadequate; total fat, saturated fat, and sodium are high; and fiber is insufficient (Kuczmarski 1998). These common dietary faults are major risk factors for chronic degenerative disorders.

Dietary intervention would be appropriate for many of these older women. Many display a willingness to improve their diets. For instance, some spoke of their efforts to meet the "5 A Day" fruit and vegetable challenge. Improved nutrient intakes can decrease risk in this age group. In a clinically controlled trial, women with a mean age of 84 years who took supplements of calcium and vitamin D experienced fewer osteoporotic fractures than women who did not take supplements (Meunier 1995). Evidence is also accumulating that women over 70 with a high total/HDL ratio benefit from dietary fat and cholesterol reduction (Kannel 1995).

While life span may not be significantly extended through improved dietary patterns instituted during the later years, morbidity may be substantially reduced. Thus, quality of life is enhanced. Some simple dietary substitutions might benefit the subjects of this study:

- Whole grains to replace refined grains, especially high fiber breakfast cereals in place of regular cereals,
- Low fat spreads on toast to replace butter and margarine,
- One serving of fruit or vegetables to replace one serving of cookies,
- An additional serving of skim milk, and
- Oil to replace butter and margarine in cooking.

A decreased incidence of disease and discomfort could result which would improve the remaining years of life. An optimal diet could help these older adults to remain vigorous and independent. Chapter 7 examines the potential of nutrition-related social support to influence the quality of the food intake pattern.

CHAPTER 7
# Functional Status, Social Support and Dietary Quality

Earlier chapters have discussed the functional status of the study participants, the attributes of their nutrition-related support, and the quality of their diets. In this chapter, interrelationships between these factors are explored following the buffering model, first presented in Chapter 1.

Each constituent in the model has been reduced to a summary score to enable statistical analyses. While summary scores are necessary to permit exploration of the model, they are unable to account for all the details. Thus, summary scores are merely proxies for the underlying constructs and the relationships between the constructs.

Three analytic hypotheses have been proposed, based on the constructs, to test the buffering model.

1. Impaired functional status will have a negative effect on diet quality.
2. Enacted, nutrition-related social support will mitigate the effects of impaired functional status on diet quality.
3. Similarly, satisfaction with nutrition-related social support (*regardless of the actual level of support*) will mitigate the effects of impaired functional status on diet quality.

Described below are the analytic methods used to test the hypotheses, the strengths and weaknesses of the methods, and the results.

## BUFFERING MODEL

In Chapter 1, a nutrition-specific model was proposed showing the associations between social relationships and diet quality. The pictorial diagram of the model, from the discussion in the first chapter, is reproduced below in Figure 15. In this research study, only a portion of the full model was examined, specifically, the associations between social support, stress, and diet quality.

The model suggests a buffering effect of social support. That is, social support influences the relationship between stress and diet quality. The model predicts that the potentially negative impact of stress on diet is greatly alleviated when social support is extensive. The negative impact of stress is only minimally reduced when social support is negligible. Furthermore, under the situation of no stress, support has no influence on diet quality. This *buffering model*, also known as the *moderator model*, is the most frequently investigated model of social support, stress, and various measures of well being (Barrera 1986; Wheaton 1985).

Figure 15: Proposed model of the association between social relationships and dietary quality (adapted from Rook 1985)

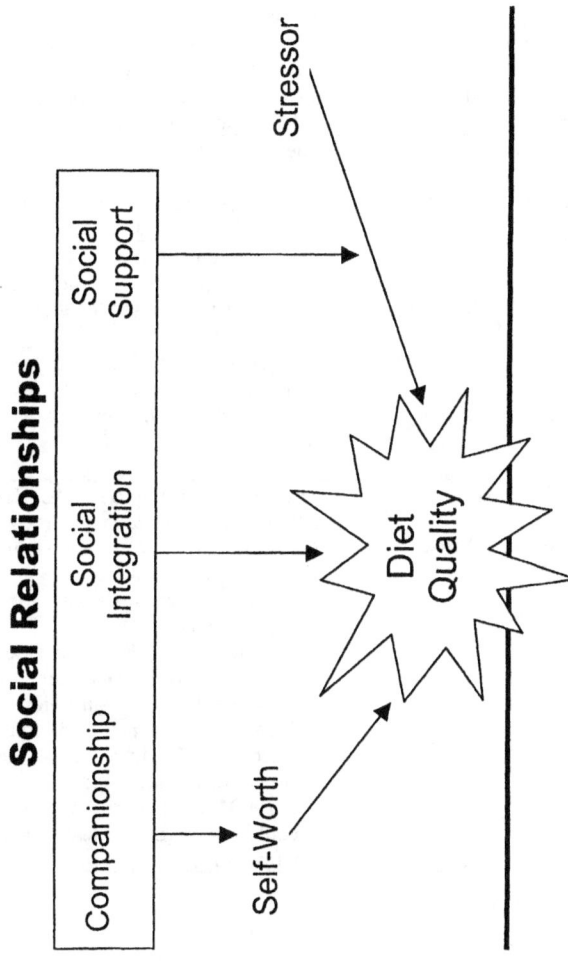

**Table 37: Brief summary of the operational definitions of dependent and independent variables**

| Variables | Operational Definition |
|---|---|
| **Food Acquisition Support** | Help with grocery shopping, including transportation, accompaniment, or actual purchase of small or large amounts of foods at the grocery store. |
| Number of helpers<br><br>Sample range = 0 to 5<br>Mean = 1.3 | The total number of helpers providing food acquisition support. (Each helper could provide more than one type of help, but is only included once in this score.) |
| Number of types<br><br>Sample range = 0 to 5<br>Mean = 1.6 | The total number of types of help being provided for food acquisition. (Each type could be provided by more than one helper, but is only included once in this score.) |
| Total helpers + types<br><br>Sample range = 0 to 10<br>Mean = 2.0 | The total number of types across all helpers for food acquisition. (Includes the total number of helpers and the total types of help in a summary score.) |
| Satisfaction<br><br>Sample range = 3 to 4<br>Mean = 3.2 | Subjects rated satisfaction as "*I need*: 1= *much less help*, 2=*a little less help*, 3=*satisfied*, 4=*a little more help*, or 5 = *much more help.*" |
| **Functional Status**<br><br>Sample range = 1 to 4<br>Mean = 2.2 | Assessed according to BADL (Katz et al. 1963), IADL (Lawton and Brody 1969) and AADL (Nagi 1976) abilities. Four levels of disability were identified –<br>  4. *None* – individuals with no impairments,<br>  3. *AADL disabilities* – individuals with at least one AADL impairment, but no IADL or BADL impairments,<br>  2. *IADL disabilities* – individuals with at least one IADL impairment, but no BADL disabilities, and,<br>  1. *BADL disabilities* – individuals who could not perform at least one BADL without help. |

| Variables | Operational Definition |
|---|---|
| **Diet Quality** | Derived from analysis of the NCI food frequency questionnaire (Block et al. 1986). |
| Diet Quality Index (DQI)<br><br>Sample range = 2 to 12<br>Mean = 6.4 | Summary score based on the 1989 National Academy of Sciences recommendations in *Diet and Health* (Patterson, Haines, and Popkin 1994). Eight dimensions are rated – percent fat, percent saturated fat, cholesterol, fruit & vegetable intake, complex carbohydrate servings, protein, sodium, and calcium. Potential range = 0 to 16. |
| Mean Adequacy Ratio (MAR)<br><br>Sample range = 50.3 to 100<br>Mean = 81.9 | Summary score based on nutrient adequacy (Guthrie and Scheer 1981). MAR is the average of the ratio of 11 nutrients relative to the RDA of each (truncated at 100% RDA). The 11 nutrients included protein, vitamin A, thiamin, riboflavin, folacin, vitamin B6, vitamin C, calcium, magnesium, iron and zinc. |

To examine the buffering model within a nutrition-specific framework, functional status was identified as one potential stressor on diet quality. The focus group participants had described the negative impact of physical disabilities on aspects of both food acquisition and food preparation. Social support was operationally defined as the number of helpers, the number of types of help, and the satisfaction with help in food acquisition.[1] Diet quality was assessed in terms of nutrients (MAR) and dietary guidelines (DQI). In earlier chapters, the calculations of each of these measures were described in detail. Table 37 contains a brief summary of the operational definitions.

All variables were considered continuous. While the operational measure of satisfaction is categorical, the underlying construct was envisioned as continuous. Similarly, functional status could be construed as categorical. However, functional status was expected to operate with social support in a continuous manner on diet quality. Statistically, the effects of functional status and social support were expected to present either as parallel lines or as a fan when graphed. No one level of function could operate in a manner disparate to the other levels.

Below is a simplified diagram of the buffering model used in this study.

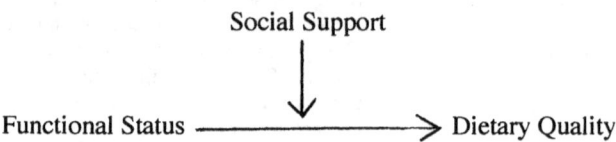

The equation used to describe the relationships between these three variables is:

Diet Quality = Functional Status + Social Support + (Functional Status x Social Support).

(The statistical equation is explained in greater detail later.)

The multiplicative term, (Functional Status x Social Support), assesses the joint influence of the two variables on diet. Essentially, the statistical significance of this variable indicates whether or not buffering effects are being detected. If the product term is significant, the buffering model is upheld. Functional status and social support are considered conditional effects – the influence of one is conditional upon the status of the other (Aiken and West 1991).

Previously the product term has been referred to as an interaction effect in both nonexperimental and experimental research. However, Pedhazur (1997) suggests the term *joint relation* in nonexperimental work. His rational is that the interpretation of joint relations differs from that of statistical interactions. In comparison to variables in experimental research, variables in nonexperimental studies usually contain more measurement error, are intercorrelated and are likely to be correlated with relevant exogenous variables (specification error). Thus, interpretation of joint relations is complex.

Note that the buffering model does not specify a direct effect of social support on diet quality. The significance of the joint relation term signifies whether functional status and social support operate synergistically or not. Investigating the main effect of social support on diet quality is inappropriate for this model.

# RELATIONSHIPS BETWEEN FUNCTIONAL STATUS, SOCIAL SUPPORT AND DIETARY QUALITY

The relationships between variables were investigated using correlation and ordinary least squares regression. The distributions of all variables were examined first. Some skewness and kurtosis was evident on all variables. Transformations were attempted. The use of a square root transformation improved the distribution of total helpers + types. The distributions of other variables showed no improvement with transformation. Thus, all variable scores remain in their raw form in the statistical analyses, except total helpers + types.

Next, diagnostics were examined (Pedhazur 1997; SAS 1996; Tabachnick and Fidell 1989). The scores of one subject exerted extreme influence on the regression equations (Mahalonobis distance at p<.0005) and were excluded from further analyses.[2]

Diagnostics continued to be evaluated during subsequent statistical analyses. Leverage and influence statistics were monitored, as well as scatter plots and residuals plots. No further cases were deleted. Thus, the sample for statistical analyses consisted of 101 elderly women. Continued inspection of diagnostics and plots aided interpretation of results.

## Functional Status and Diet Quality

The first research hypothesis to be tested examined the relationship between functional status and dietary quality. Functional impairments were hypothesized to be associated with a diet of lower quality. However, Pearson correlation coefficients showed no relationship between functional status and DQI (r=.03, p=.77) nor functional status and MAR (r=.09, p=.38).

Other researchers have found significant relationships between functional status and dietary quality in their samples (Bianchetti et al. 1990; Hunter and Linn 1979; Walker and Beauchene 1991). Some of the difference in findings is attributable to differences in the operational definitions of functional status and diet quality. For instance, Hunter and Linn (1979) found a correlation of .22 (p<.05) between a measure of physical disability and a food group score in 88 older adults.

Walker and Beauchene (1991) reported a correlation of .28 between MAR and a Gutman-ranked BADL score in 61 elders. In comparison, the subjects in this study can be divided into two groups—those who have difficulty with BADL activities and those who do not. Using these categories, a Spearman correlation coefficient of .19 (p=.06) exists between functional status and MAR. The individuals with BADL difficulties have a mean MAR score of 78.8 in comparison to 83.5 for individuals with no BADL disabilities ($t=-1.7$, p=.08). No correlation exists between BADL disabilities and DQI.

Bianchetti et al. (1990) examined nutrient intakes and IADL disabilities using chi-square analyses. They reported that individuals who had lost one or more IADL capabilities were more likely to have poor nutrient intakes. This research sample can also be divided into individuals with and without IADL disabilities. Again, a significant Spearman correlation of .22 (p=.02) exists between MAR and IADL capabilities. Individuals who are incapable of performing one or more IADL activities have a mean MAR score of 74.6 in comparison to 83.1 for individuals with no IADL disabilities ($t=-2.38$, p=.02). No correlation exists between IADL disabilities and DQI.

In summary, when older adults have difficulty with Basic Activities of Daily Living or are unable to perform Instrumental Activities of Daily Living, nutrient intake appears compromised. However, even minor losses in functional status are expected to influence food patterns (Dwyer 1991). Yet no relationship was found between the broader scale assessing advanced, instrumental, and basic ADLs and either measure of diet quality (MAR and DQI). The lack of a relationship can be attributed to:

- measurement error,
- true fluctuations in the functional status of individuals (Crimmins and Saito 1993), and
- exogenous variables and joint relations that are simultaneously influencing diet quality.

Although the relationship between functional status and diet quality was not statistically significant in this study, the possibility of a joint relation with social support remains. In the next section the buffering model is investigated.

## Functional Status, Social Support and Diet Quality

As previously discussed ordinary least squares regression was used to examine the joint relations of functional status and social support on dietary quality (Cohen and Wills 1985; Wheaton 1985). The multiple regression equation took the form:

$$Y = b_0 + b_1 X + b_2 Z + b_3 XZ + \varepsilon$$

where
- $X$ = Functional Status
- $Z$ = Social Support
- $XZ$ = Joint Relation (Functional Status x Social Support)
- $Y$ = Dietary Quality
- $b_0$ = intercept
- $b_1$ to $b_3$ = partial regression coefficients
- $\varepsilon$ = error

Three summary scores exist for enacted social support

- number of helpers,
- number of types and
- total helpers + types.

Two summary scores were evaluated for dietary quality

- MAR and
- DQI.

Thus, a number of regression series were examined to investigate the second analytic hypothesis—that enacted, nutrition-related social support will mitigate the effects of impaired functional status on diet quality.

*The influence of functional status, number of helpers, and the joint relation on Diet Quality Index*

Hierarchical regression has been recommended to ensure that the equation containing the joint term explains more variance than simpler models (McClelland and Judd 1993; Pedhazur 1997). Table 38 shows the results of a hierarchical regression series with DQI as the outcome variable and functional status and number of helpers as the independent variables.

**Table 38: Hierarchical regression results examining the influence of functional status, numbers of helpers and the joint relation on DQI. Independent variables are centered**

| Equation | constant | Outcome = DQI | | | Adj. $R^2$ |
| | | $b_1$ Functional Status | $b_2$ Number of Helpers | $b_3$ Funtional Status x Number of Helpers | |
|---|---|---|---|---|---|
| 1 | 6.396 | 0.070 | | | -0.009 |
| 2 | 6.396 | -0.242 | -0.610* | | 0.039♦ |
| 3 | 6.091 | -0.417 | -0.760** | -0.558* | 0.083** |

♦ $p<.10$
\* $p<.05$
\*\* $p<.01$

Independent variables are centered (subtracted from the mean) to improve interpretation of first order effects (Aiken and West 1991). Uncentered values lead to highly unstable regression coefficients of the first order terms due to multicollinearity between variables. Centered and uncentered equations have identical regression slopes and significance tests of the joint relation term. Finney et al., (1984) point out that centering permits estimation of averaged conditional effects. That is, the conditional effect of functional status at the average level of social support can be derived, as well as the conditional effect of social support at the average level of functional status.

Table 38 shows that the joint relation of functional status and number of helpers significantly predicts DQI. As the main effect model falls short of statistical significance, the product term appears essential to the equation. A global test is available to test the significance of the gain in prediction (Aiken and West 1991; Dunlap and Kemery 1988).

$$F = \frac{(R^2\text{in} - R^2\text{out})/m}{(1 \pm R^2\text{in})/(n - k - 1)} \qquad df = m, (n-k-1)$$

where   $R^2$in = squared multiple correlation of joint equation
$R^2$out = squared multiple correlation of main effects equation
m = number terms that differ between equations
n = number of subjects
k = number of predictors in joint equation.

The results of the global test indicate that the joint equation for DQI significantly enhances prediction over the main effects model (F=4.76, p<.05, $df$=1,97).

Figure 16 is a graphical display of the joint relation effects of functional status and number of helpers on DQI. For individuals with no functional impairments, the influence of help is very strong. For fully functional elders, the equation predicts an improvement of $1^3/_4$ points to the DQI score with each additional helper. The scores of women with AADL disabilities improve $1^1/_4$ points with the addition of each helper. Women with IADL disabilities realize less improvement, 2/3 point per additional helper. For women with BADL disabilities, additional help is not indicative of any change in DQI.

**Table 39: Simple slope analysis results at each level of functional ability, for the equation DQI = Functional Status + Number of Helpers + Joint Relation.**

| Disability Level | b | SE b | T | Sig T |
| --- | --- | --- | --- | --- |
| BADL | -0.098 | 0.323 | -0.302 | 0.7630 |
| IADL | -0.655 | 0.246 | -2.667 | 0.0090 |
| AADL | -1.213 | 0.351 | -3.451 | 0.0008 |
| None | -1.771 | 0.542 | -3.266 | 0.0015 |

The statistical significance of the simple slope at each level of functional status can be determined by t-tests. Table 39 shows that the simple slope of the regression line for BADL impaired women does not differ from zero. That is, additional help is not associated with better diet quality for women with BADL disabilities. The statistical significance of the simple slope for IADL disabled subjects appears somewhat questionable when looking at Figure 16. The results of the t-test clarify that additional help is associated with significantly better diet quality for women with IADL disabilities. Additional help is also associated with significantly better diets for women with AADL disabilities or no disabilities.

Figure 16 clearly demonstrates the meaning of the joint relation. Without knowing the level of functional status, the influence of help on DQI can not be predicted. In reverse, without knowing the level of help, the impact of functional status on DQI can not be elucidated. The statistical significance of the joint relation term indicates that the slopes of the lines differ across levels of functional status (Aiken and West 1991). In other words, no additional statistical tests are needed to determine if the simple slope of the regression line for BADL disabled differs from the simple slope for IADL disabled, AADL disabled, or not disabled.

In interpreting the joint relation between functional status and number of helpers, the correlation between the two variables must also be considered. In this sample of women the Pearson correlation coefficient equals -.49 (p=.0001). Poorer functional status is significantly related to a greater number of helpers. Figure 17 shows the average number of helpers at each level of functional status.

☐ In a statistical sense, a correlation of -.49 is considered moderate and serves to underscore the previous point by Pedhazur (1997). Statistical interaction refers to a joint effect of unrelated variables. However, in a practical sense, the correlation emphasizes the need to simultaneously consider both functional status and social support. Every individual with poor functional status does not have a large number of helpers.

In summary, the joint relation of functional status and the number of helpers with food acquisition has a statistically significant effect on DQI. The diets of women with no disabilities show the most improvement with the addition of each helper. However, women with no disabilities are the least likely to receive help. At the other extreme, the diets of women with BADL disabilities show no improvement as the number of helpers increase. Additional help is not associated with any change in the quality of the diet. The diets of women with AADL and IADL disabilities fall between the extremes.

**Figure 16: Graph showing the joint relation of functional status and number of helpers on Diet Quality Index**

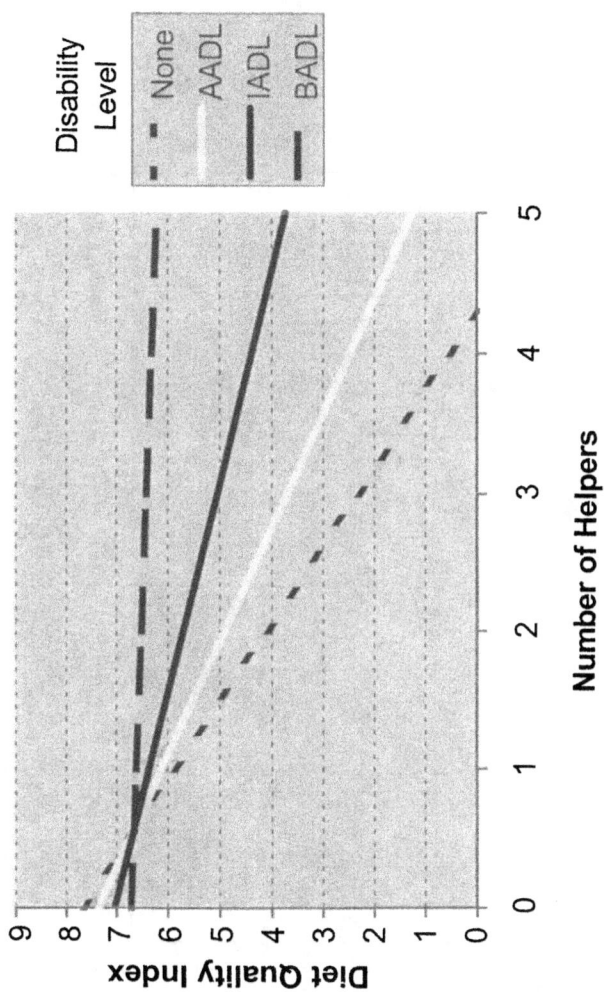

**Figure 17: Mean helpers + SD by functional status**

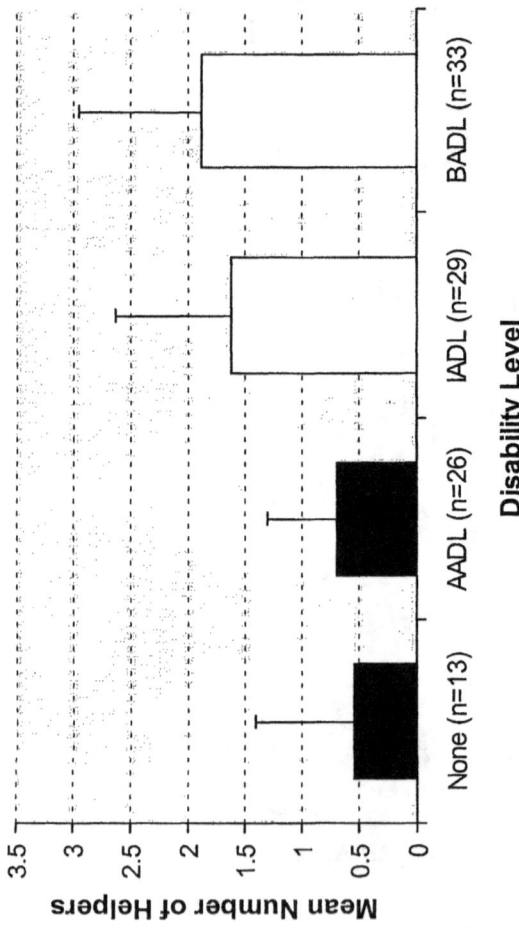

Note: Results of PROC GLM indicate that the mean number of helpers differs between groups (F=11.82, p<.0001). Values of black and white bars significantly different.

## The influence of functional status, number of helpers, and the joint relation on Mean Adequacy Ratio

Clearly, a joint effect is influencing the healthfulness of the diet in comparison to the dietary guidelines. However, do functional status and number of helpers influence the nutrient content of the diet in the same manner? DQI and MAR are moderately correlated with a Pearson correlation coefficient of .39 ($p<.0001$). While somewhat related, the scores are obviously measuring different dimensions of the diet. Table 40 shows the results of the hierarchical regression series for MAR.

According to strict statistical criteria, the joint relation of functional status and number of helpers falls short of significance at $p=.126$. However, examination of regression line plots and alternative graphs, such as Figure 18, suggest a synergistic relationship between functional status and number of helpers on MAR.

**Table 40: Hierarchical regression results examining the influence of functional status, number of helpers and the joint relation on MAR. Independent variables are centered.**

| | Outcome = MAR | | | | |
|---|---|---|---|---|---|
| Equation | constant | $b_1$ Functional Status | $b_2$ Number of Helpers | $b_3$ Funtional Status x Number of Helpers | Adj. $R^2$ |
| 1 | 81.995 | 1.084 | | | -0.002 |
| 2 | 81.925 | 3.027* | 3.780** | | 0.067* |
| 3 | 82.960 | 3.622* | 4.305** | 1.894 | 0.080* |

* $p<.05$
** $p<.01$

In Figure 18 note how the MAR score improves within functional status categories as the number of helpers increases. In contrast, the MAR score decreases when the functional status category declines but the number of helpers remains consistent. This decreasing trend is especially apparent within the group of women receiving help from one person.

**Figure 18: Average Mean Adequacy Ratio (MAR) by number of helpers and functional status**

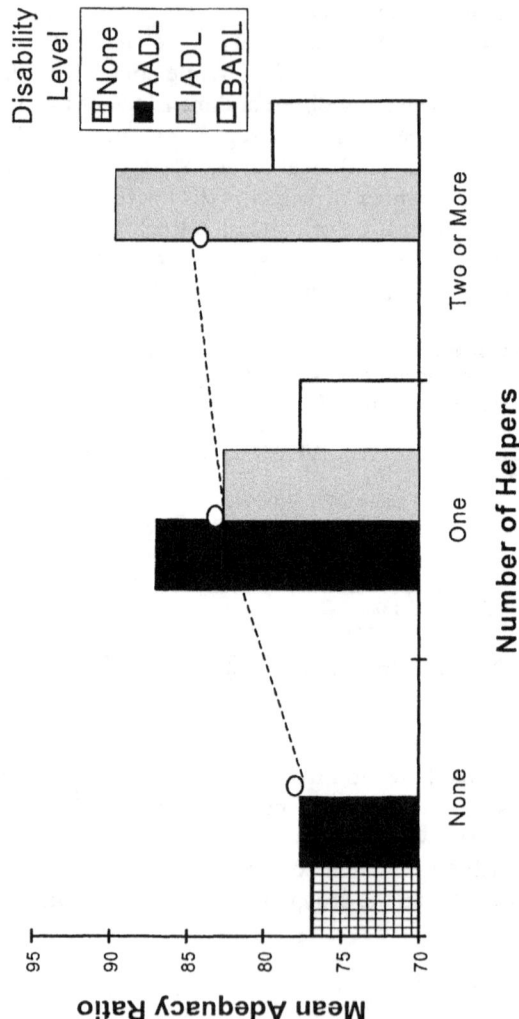

Note: The bars are displayed only for groups with five or more members. The average MAR of groups with less than five members may be misleading. Thus the MARs of 92 project participants are included on the bar charts; 101 participants are included in the overall means for the three levels of help (ovals and dashed line).

## Conclusions

In nonexperimental research, moderated regression often fails to detect expected joint relations (McClelland and Judd 1993). Yet, in experimental situations, moderated regression is a powerful tool. Statistical power is reduced in nonexperimental studies for several reasons (Aiken and West 1991; McClelland and Judd 1993).

- Measurement error—error in assessment of the first order terms is amplified in the cross product term.
- Unknown exogenous effects—model misspecification is similarly magnified in the cross product term.
- Restricted range—limitations in the theoretical range of the cross product reduce the possibility of detecting a significant effect.
- Nonlinearity—mild curvilinear trends further weaken the power of moderated regression.
- Residual variance—mid-range scores and the pairing of mid-range with extreme scores decrease residual variance and thus, efficiency of moderated regression.

Most of these reasons for decreased power are recognized attributes of the nonexperimental method. Field researchers attempt to optimize measurement reliability and model specificity, and to decrease other sources of error. However, the complexity of the real-world situation often dictates unknowns into the model.

McClelland and Judd (1993) recommend three options to enhance detection of joint effects in nonexperimental situations:

1. accept a higher Type I error rate,
2. increase sample size,
3. oversample extreme values.

None of the options is without criticism. If option 1 is implemented, confidence in the results is decreased. The required sample size for option 2 is "*enormous*" according to McClelland and Judd (1993). Option 3 biases results and reduces generalizability of the findings.

In the case of this research project, increasing the risk of Type I error to reduce the chance of Type II error appears to be a viable option.[3] The p value of the joint relation is .126. Figure 18 certainly suggests a joint relation between functional status and number of helpers. Furthermore, examining the residuals from the full equation shows that the joint relation term is compromised by unexpectedly low MAR scores of two women. Both women are high functioning and receive high levels of help, but nonetheless have diets of poor quality. If they are dropped from the equation, the joint relation term is statistically significant at $p=.034$. The equation explains 12% of the variance in MAR at $p=.002$.

These two women do appear members of the population under study and should not be omitted from the analyses. The results are reported here merely to emphasize the fragility of the joint relation term in the nonexperimental situation.

A joint effect of functional status and number of helpers on MAR is supported by additional analyses. One weakness of the MAR score is a high association with caloric intake (Kant 1996). In this sample, MAR and total calories have a Pearson correlation of 0.73, $p<.0001$. Under-reporting and over-reporting on the food frequency questionnaire would influence MAR. The large range of caloric intake in this study (557 to 2567 calories/day) does suggest under- and over-estimates of average daily intakes. Thus, nutrient density rather than absolute nutrient intake may be a better indicator of diet quality.

Total caloric intake per day can be added to the moderated regression equation as a control variable. Results are shown in Table 41. As expected, caloric intake accounts for a significant percentage of the variation in MAR score. When functional status or number of helpers are added, no main effects are seen.

## Conclusions

**Table 41: Hierarchical regression results examining the influence of average calories per day, functional status, number of helpers and the joint relation of functional status x number of helpers on MAR. Independent variables are centered.**

| | | Outcome = MAR | | | | |
|---|---|---|---|---|---|---|
| Equation | constant | $b_1$ Calories/ Day | $b_2$ Functional Status | $b_3$ Number of Helpers | $b_4$ Funtional Status x Number of Helpers | Adj. $R^2$ |
| 1 | 81.925 | 0.022*** | | | | 0.524*** |
| 2 | 81.925 | 0.022*** | 0.276 | | | 0.520*** |
| 3 | 81.925 | 0.021*** | 1.060 | 1.469 | | 0.526*** |
| 4 | 82.918 | 0.021*** | 1.636 | 1.976* | 1.818* | 0.543*** |

\* p<.05
\*\*\* p<.0001

However, the joint term is statistically significant. The predictive potential of the equation, assessed by the increase in $R^2$, does not reach statistical significance as evaluated by the global test described earlier (F=1.33, p=ns, $df$=3,96). Regardless, the main reason for running this regression series was to evaluate the effects of the joint relation. The results demonstrate that after MAR has been adjusted for caloric intake, the joint effect of functional status and number of helpers contributes to the model.

McClelland and Judd (1993) report that in nonexperimental situations, joint relations typically account for only 1–3% of the variance. These authors contend that field studies finding an effect size as little as 1% attributable to the joint relation have much practical significance. McClelland and Judd use a case study to demonstrate that 1% in a field study is equivalent to about 22% in an optimal experimental situation.

Figure 19 shows the joint relation effects of functional status and number of helpers on MAR. Except for the reverse scoring of MAR and DQI, the graph looks quite similar to Figure 16. For individuals with no functional disabilities, MAR increases $5^1/_4$ points with the addition of each helper. In contrast, for individuals with BADL disabilities, MAR shows no change at different levels of help. The MAR scores of

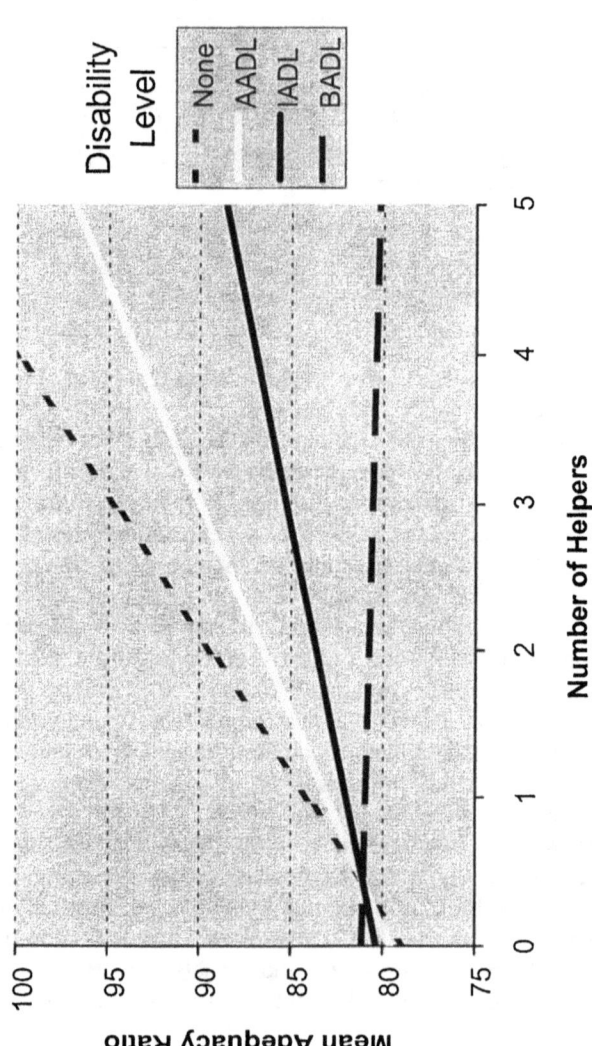

**Figure 19:** Graph showing the joint relation of functional status and number of helpers on Mean Adequacy Ratio while controlling for caloric intake

women with IADL and AADL disabilities fall between the two extremes.

Again, the statistical significance of the simple slope at each level of functional status was determined. The results are shown in Table 42. In contrast to the results with DQI, the slopes for both BADL and IADL disability levels do not differ from zero. In other words, for women with BADL or IADL impairments additional helpers are not indicative of any change in nutrient quality. However, the diets of women with AADL or no disabilities are significantly better for women who receive help from more individuals.

**Table 42: Simple slope analysis results at each level of functional ability, for the equation MAR = Calories/Day + Functional Status + Number of Helpers + Joint Relation of Functional Status x Number of Helpers**

| Disability Level | b      | SE b  | T      | Sig T |
|------------------|--------|-------|--------|-------|
| BADL             | -0.184 | 1.230 | -0.150 | 0.881 |
| IADL             | 1.634  | 0.948 | 1.724  | 0.088 |
| AADL             | 3.452  | 1.336 | 2.584  | 0.011 |
| None             | 5.271  | 2.043 | 2.580  | 0.011 |

In summary, results of moderated regression suggest that the joint relation of functional status and number of helpers influences dietary quality, whether diet quality is assessed according to nutrient content or according to the dietary guidelines. The effect of functional status is conditional on the number of helpers; and vice versa, the effect of the number of helpers is conditional on the level of functional status.

**Alternative measures of food acquisition support**

Alternative measures of nutrition-related social support were also investigated in the buffering model. Tables 43 and 44 show the results. The joint relation terms were not statistically significant in any of the equations. The results appear to indicate that neither the number of types nor the total helpers + types moderates the impact of functional status on diet quality.

**Table 43: Hierarchical regression results examining the influence of functional status, number of types of help and the joint relation on diet quality. Independent variables are centered.**

|  | constant | $b_1$ Functional Status | $b_2$ No. of Types of Help | $b_3$ Functional Status x No. of Types of Help | Adj. $R^2$ |
|---|---|---|---|---|---|
| Equation | | | Outcome = DQI | | |
| 1 | 6.396 | 0.070 | | | -0.009 |
| 2 | 6.396 | -0.005 | -0.147 | | -0.015 |
| 3 | 6.136 | -0.191 | -0.170 | -0.481* | 0.018 |
| Equation | | | Outcome = MAR | | |
| 1 | 81.925 | 1.084 | | | -0.002 |
| 2 | 81.925 | 1.816 | 1.442 | | 0.004 |
| 3 | 83.193 | 2.726♦ | 1.554 | 2.349♦ | 0.030 |

♦ p<.10
* p<.05

Number of types of help may not be an optimal measure to evaluate social support in this situation. Types of food acquisition support may be substituted rather than added. For most individuals, as functional status declines, the number of types of help increases. The two variables were negatively associated with a Pearson correlation coefficient of -.43 (p<.0001). However, at the lowest levels of functioning, going out to the grocery store may not be possible. Thus, the full range of types of help is not available. Figure 20 shows that the mean number of types of help slightly decreased from the level of IADL disabled to BADL disabled.

In addition, the lack of significant findings in Tables 43 and 44 may be attributable to the limitations of moderated regression with nonexperimental research. The p values for the full model equations of Tables 43 and 44 ranged from .05 to .19. The p values for the joint relation terms ranged from .04 to .13. Considering that number of helpers and functional status do exert a joint effect on diet quality, further exploratory work using these measures appeared warranted.

**Table 44: Hierarchical regression results examining the influence of functional status, total helpers + types of help and the joint relation on diet quality. Independent variables are centered.**

|  | constant | $b_1$ Functional Status | $b_2$ Total Helpers + Types[a] | $b_3$ Functional Status x Total Helpers + Types[a] | Adj. $R^2$ |
|---|---|---|---|---|---|
| Equation | | Outcome = DQI | | | |
| 1 | 6.396 | 0.070 | | | -0.009 |
| 2 | 6.396 | -0.173 | -0.604 | | 0.008 |
| 3 | 6.166 | -0.270 | -0.544 | -0.540♦ | 0.025 |
| Equation | | Outcome = MAR | | | |
| 1 | 81.925 | 1.084 | | | -0.002 |
| 2 | 81.925 | 2.826♦ | 4.346* | | 0.038♦ |
| 3 | 83.026 | 3.293* | 4.055* | 2.583 | 0.051* |

[a] The scores are transformed with the square root to improve distribution.
♦ p<.10
** p<.05

Examination of residuals suggested the possibility of curvilinear trends. A quadratic social support term and a quadratic joint relation term were added to the model (Aiken and West 1991):

Diet Quality = Functional Status + Social Support + (Social Support)$^2$ + (Functional Status)(Social Support) + (Functional Status)(Social Support)$^2$.

The curvilinear equation was statistically significant for both DQI equations. However, graphing of the results showed overfitting of the data. Specifically two individuals with AADL disabilities and high levels of help were creating the need for the curvilinear fit.

McClelland and Judd (1993) point out that the mathematical computations of moderated regression rely on extreme cases to detect joint effects. In this investigation, high functioning women with high levels of help and low functioning women with no help are poorly represented. In fact, no one without disability receives help from three or more individuals. At the opposite extreme, only two women with BADL disabilities receive no help at all.

**Figure 20: Mean types of help + SD by functional status**

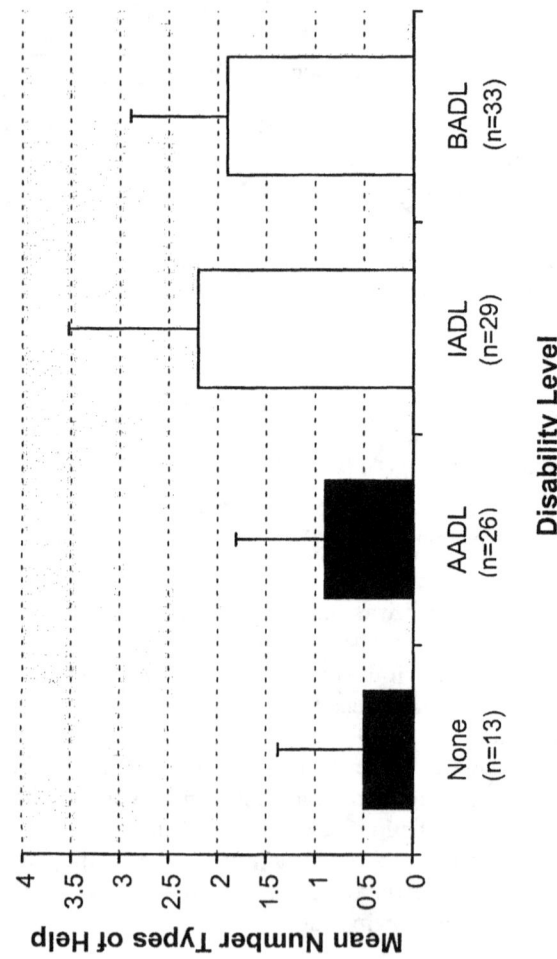

Note: Results of PROC GLM indicate that the mean number of helpers differs between groups (F=11.82, p<.0001). Values of black and white bars significantly different.

Conclusions 163

Thus, the results of Tables 43 and 44 remain in question. The suggestions of McClelland and Judd (1993) on page 155 are again relevant. The findings would be more convincing if the sample contained a larger number of women in the extreme categories of social support. Interviewing more women in the extremes would mean either oversampling those categories or recruiting a huge number of participants. Greater numbers would enhance confidence in the results. No longer would significance depend on the reliability of only a few scores.

## SATISFACTION WITH FOOD ACQUISITION SUPPORT

Satisfaction with social support is expected to moderate the relationship between stress and well being in a manner similar to enacted support (Landerman et al. 1989). An individual's evaluation of satisfaction will simultaneously balance her perceived need for support with the actual provision of support. Thus, our third analytic hypothesis stated that satisfaction with nutrition-related social support will mitigate the effects of impaired functional status on diet quality.

Two problems in measuring satisfaction with food acquisition support occurred in this study. First, as discussed in Chapter 6, one of the interviewers erroneously omitted this question for 22 respondents. Most of the women who were not asked the question had high functional status and received little or no help. Thus, the subsample for which results are available is not representative of the entire group.

Secondly, only 13 out of the 84 women who were asked about satisfaction with food acquisition replied that they would like "*a little more help*." The interview question was designed to be more sensitive—appraising feelings of over-support (controlling helpers), mild under-support, and major lack of support.

Table 45 shows the results of the hierarchical regression series examining the influence of satisfaction with food acquisition and functional status on diet quality. The uneven split (13:71) and the low number of dissatisfied women across four levels of functional status leaves little potential to detect a moderating effect. As expected, the results show no significant outcomes.

**Table 45: Hierarchical regression results examining the influence of functional status, satisfaction with food acquistion support and the joint relation on diet quality. Functional status is centered.**

|  | constant | $b_1$ Functional Status | $b_2$ Satisfaction | $b_3$ Functional Status x Satisfaction | Adj. $R^2$ |
|---|---|---|---|---|---|
| Equation | | | Outcome = DQI | | |
| 1 | 6.247 | -0.161 | | | -0.008 |
| 2 | 5.031 | -0.154 | 0.386 | | -0.017 |
| 3 | 4.988 | -0.334 | 0.400 | 0.057 | -0.029 |
| Equation | | | Outcome = MAR | | |
| 1 | 82.939 | 1.833 | | | 0.007 |
| 2 | 70.896 | 1.898 | 3.821 | | 0.007 |
| 3 | 75.696 | 21.898♦ | 2.272 | -6.317 | 0.027 |

♦ $p < .10$

## DISCUSSION

In light of the limitations of moderated regression in nonexperimental research, the results appear to favor a buffering effect of nutrition-related social support on the relationship between functional status and dietary quality. The number of providers of social support was a better predictor of diet quality than the number of types of social support. Types may be substitutive rather than additive.

Unfortunately, this study lacked an effective measure of the perceived quality of support. Either the questionnaire item was ineffective in tapping the true feelings of the subjects, or many of the women feel that a low level of support is adequate. Krause (1989) has suggested that the ideal of reciprocity may influence the evaluation of adequacy. He posits that the inability of older adults to reciprocate leads them to prefer minimal levels of help. The alternative would be to admit an unequal relationship or dependency. Many of the elderly subjects in this study stated that they are unable to furnish much help to others at this stage in their lives.

Thus, the findings of this study are limited to enacted, instrumental, nutrition-related social support and the joint effect with functional status on diet quality in elderly women living in government subsidized housing. Women with few disabilities who receive help from many sources have a diet of better quality in comparison to women who receive help from few sources. Receiving even a small amount of support in obtaining foods, for example having someone pick up milk or orange juice a few times a month, appears related to a more healthful diet for women with high functional capabilities. However, women with few disabilities are unlikely to obtain even this small amount of aid.

At the opposite extreme, the dietary quality of women with many disabilities who receive help from many sources is similar to the dietary quality of women who receive help from few sources. Again, the ideal of reciprocity may be influential. Perhaps the women accept only a minimum level of needed help because they are unable to reciprocate. That is, they only accept enough help to permit maintenance of a marginally sufficient diet. Alternatively, health problems, control issues, or other influences may be simultaneously affecting diet quality.

In conclusion, the results suggest that the diets of women under little or no nutrition stress are better when instrumental support is perceived. The diets of women under severe stress are similar across levels of instrumental help. The results also suggest that these effects are apparent with as little as one helper, but are more pronounced at two or more helpers.

The results prompt a number of intriguing questions. Are there other differences between the mildly and not disabled women who receive help and those who do not receive help? Would a simple intervention, such as a three item grocery delivery service, make a difference in overall diet quality? For women with moderate to severe disabilities, if additional instrumental support does not improve diet quality, what might be beneficial? Would the removal of an existing support cause a decline in diet quality? What are the longitudinal effects?

Obviously, additional research is necessary to further delineate the influence of functional status and food acquisition support on diet quality. Furthermore, additional research is needed to examine other sources of nutrition stress, other forms of social support on diet, and other population groups.

## NOTES

1. Summary scores including meal preparation statistics were also explored. Initial analyses suggested few inter-relationships between diet quality, functional status, and meal preparation support. A number of factors contributed to the poor associations. Following are a few reasons why scoring methods including meal acquisition statistics appeared inappropriate for the desired analyses.
    a. Assessment questions had overlooked meals eaten in food service establishments. Some children frequently took their mother out to eat, rather than prepare a home-cooked meal.
    b. Gifts of food were too variable in their nutritional content, ranging from small quantities to full meals.
    c. In-home food preparation and home-delivered meals were only used by a small minority of subjects, and did not contribute sufficiently to the scores.

Use of congregate meals was examined in depth and demonstrated no relationship to diet quality or functional status.

2. The subject was a multivariate outlier due to the simultaneous conditions of very high support, AADL disabilities, and a diet of average quality. Katherine stated that she walks to the grocery store with three friends every day. Furthermore, her son drives her to a grocery store once each week and her daughter occasionally brings requested groceries. Her reported diet averages 808 calories/day, with a DQI of 6 and an MAR of 67. Her BMI is 41.

Her situation is unique based on the statistical combination of all three factors. Most likely one of her scores is imprecise. The high BMI and low caloric intake suggest that the dietary information may be inaccurate. Alternatively, her level of help may have been incorrectly classified. Perhaps the three friends should have been coded as one source of help. Furthermore, the statistical method does not permit curvilinear trends. Katherine's combination of scores might not be as extreme if predicted diet quality tapered at high levels of function and support.

3. Type I error is the risk of rejecting a true hypothesis. In this case, concluding that functional status and number of helpers do influence diet quality when in fact, they do not. Type II error is the risk of not rejecting a false hypothesis. In this case, concluding that functional status and number of helpers do not have a joint effect on diet quality when in fact, they do. By decreasing Type II error, statistical power is always increased (Tabachnick and Fidell 1989).

CHAPTER 8
# Conclusions

The purpose of this research project was to provide descriptive information on the functions and providers of nutrition-related social support, and to examine the effects of functional status and nutrition-related social support on diet quality. Previous chapters have explored the findings in detail. In this concluding chapter, a brief summary of the results is presented.

The findings for each of the originally proposed descriptive outcomes and analytic research hypotheses are described in a condensed format. The results are considered with respect to the model of social relationships and diet quality presented in Chapter 1. In addition, the limitations of the research methodology are discussed, as well as generalizability of the findings. Recommendations for policy and program initiatives are considered. Finally, suggestions for related future research are outlined.

## SUMMARY OF RESULTS

In brief, four focus groups, 12 key informant interviews, and 102 structured interviews were conducted. The primary objective of the focus groups was to discern the nutrition-related concerns of elderly women. Through the key informant interviews the types of support offered in response to the identified problems were distinguished. The 102 structured interviews provided descriptive information on the frequency of providers and types of support in a larger sample. The collections of qualitative and quantitative data were analyzed to meet specific research outcomes and hypotheses, detailed below.

## Descriptive Outcomes

*Outcome 1: A classification scheme of nutrition-related helping behaviors, as reported by older women, will be developed.*

A classification scheme of nutrition-related helping behaviors was developed from the results of the 12 key informant interviews. Four categories of help were identified, including instrumental, informational, emotional, and availability. Instrumental help includes food preparation, grocery shopping, providing transportation, and accompaniment to the grocery store. Informational help includes advice, education, and direction. Emotional help includes encouragement and self-disclosure. Availability refers to the accessibility of the helper, most typically in conjunction with the provision of instrumental types of aid.

Other researchers have examined the helping behaviors perceived by low-income, young mothers (Gottlieb 1978), filial caregivers (Abel 1989), and cancer victims (Dakof and Taylor 1990). The categories of nutrition-related social support were similar to the categories of support offered to these other groups. Both similarities and differences are apparent in the specific types of support offered to the elderly women of this study in comparison to the young mothers, the caregivers, and the cancer victims. The findings uphold the principle that social support is specific to the situation and to the interpersonal relationships involved in the situation.

*Outcome 2: The frequency of instrumental, informational, and emotional social support functions will be examined in response to identified food and nutrition problems of elders. In addition, the providers of the various types of support will be identified.*

The discussion groups and key informant interviews were held to identify the food and nutrition problems of elderly women. The participants discussed a number of concerns with the potential to negatively impact food acquisition, food preparation, and food consumption. Two stressors, functional status and modified diets, appear to generate the most social support. Functional status influences grocery acquisition and meal preparation, while modified diets influence food consumption patterns.

Instrumental types of support are offered to help individuals acquire food and meals. Emotional and informational types of support are offered for modified diets. Overall, 97 of the 102 women reported receipt of at least one of these types of support.

Almost 90% receive instrumental types of help. In contrast, only 42% of the women following modified diets receive emotional or informational support. Women with more functional limitations receive more instrumental support. Women following physician-prescribed diets are more likely to receive emotional and informational support than are women on self-prescribed diets. However, if help is received, the number of helpers is similar regardless of diet origin.

Most of the support is received from informal sources. Friends are the most frequent providers of instrumental support, followed closely by daughters and then sons. Daughters are the most frequent providers of emotional and informational support, followed by friends. Task specificity is evident. Daughters are the primary providers of advice, encouragement and meal invitations. Friends are the primary sources of self-disclosure and gifts of food.

Fewer subjects reported help from formal sources. Thirty-six percent participate in meal programs, 17% receive help from homemaker aids, and 13% receive support from physicians. As expected, task specificity is again evident. Meal programs provide meals. Homemaker aids provide food preparation and grocery shopping help. Physicians provide encouragement and directives on following diet modifications.

In summary, the findings are in agreement with much of the related literature (Crohan and Antonucci 1989; Rook and Schuster 1996). A hierarchy of preferred support providers is evident, as well as task specificity. The majority of the support arises from informal sources, with family and friends about evenly divided. Disabled subjects are more likely to receive instrumental help from formal sources, such as home health aids and home delivered meals.

*Outcome 3: The older women's satisfaction with nutrition-related social support will be described. Again, the providers of the support will be considered simultaneously.*

The majority of the subjects indicated that they are satisfied with the support they receive. Due to interviewer error, not all women were asked the satisfaction questions. Of those who were polled, only 16% desire more help with grocery acquisition, 13% want more help with meal acquisition, and 19% desire more help following modified diets.

The correlates to wanting more help vary with the type of help desired. However, BMI showed some interesting associations. A higher BMI is related to wanting both more meal acquisition and modified diet support. Simultaneously, a higher BMI is related to the belief that prior help was ineffectual.

Level of satisfaction did not appear to be related to the relationships of the providers, the specific types of support, nor the number of helpers. However, the results from this small and nonrepresentative subsample must be interpreted with caution. Satisfaction with support has proven a simple and reliable indicator of the effectiveness of social support in other situations (Barrera 1986; Landerman et al. 1989). Further research is necessary to determine the suitability of satisfaction as an indicator of nutrition-related support.

**Analytic Research Hypotheses**

*Hypothesis 1: Impaired functional status will have a negative effect on diet quality.*

No direct association was found between the broad measure of functional status and diet quality, measured as either MAR or DQI. In contrast, prior research has documented correlations ranging from .22–.28 (Bianchetti et al. 1990; Hunter and Linn 1979; Walker and Beauchene 1991). The previous researchers defined functional status as a low level cut-point, rather than the spectrum from full functioning to low functioning, as in this study. By approximating the scoring methods of the prior studies, an association was noted between functional status and MAR, but not between functional abilities and DQI.

*Hypothesis 2: Enacted, nutrition-related social support will mitigate the effects of impaired functional status on diet quality.*

The results of moderated multiple regression indicated that the joint effect of functional status and number of helpers of grocery acquisition support on DQI was statistically significant. The diet quality of individuals with severe disabilities is similar across the number of helpers. In contrast, the diet quality of individuals with no disabilities is better if help is received from many people than if help is received from only a few people. The diet quality of women with mild and moderate impairments falls between the two extremes.

The joint effect of functional status and the number of providers of grocery acquisition support on MAR approached statistical significance. Considering the limitations of moderated regression with nonexperimental research, the findings strongly suggest that the joint effect on MAR is meaningful. Post hoc analyses demonstrated that the joint effect of functional status and number of helpers on nutrient density (MAR controlled for caloric intake) achieved statistical significance.

Social support was also defined as the number of types of grocery acquisition support and the number of helpers by types of grocery acquisition support. Neither of these measures resulted in statistically significant findings. Types of food acquisition support may be substitutive rather than additive. In particular, women with severe disabilities are unable to use some forms of support, such as accompaniment to the grocery store.

In summary, number of helpers appears to be a better indicator of nutrition-related social support than number of types. The relationship of number of helpers with functional status, $r=-.49$, must also be considered. In other words, women under little nutrition stress who receive instrumental support consume the healthiest diets. However, high functioning women are unlikely to receive help. Diet quality is reduced for women under greater stress or with fewer sources of support. Even though women with severe disabilities are more likely to receive help, diet quality remains similar regardless of the number of helpers. Issues of reciprocal balance and dependency may influence acceptance of support.

*Hypothesis 3: Similarly, satisfaction with nutrition-related social support (regardless of the actual level of support) will mitigate the effects of impaired functional status on diet quality.*

As mentioned under Outcome 3, the satisfaction question was erroneously omitted from some interviews. Moreover, the questionnaire item did not appear very sensitive. None of the subjects reported misguided support nor major lack of support. Only 13 individuals stated that they would like *"a little more help."* Not surprisingly, the results of moderated regression showed no statistically significant joint effect of satisfaction and functional status on diet quality.

## Synopsis

The results indicate that nutrition-related social support includes emotional, informational, and instrumental types of help. Both types of help and providers of help vary with the source of nutrition stress. Emotional and informational types of support, such as reassurance, encouragement, and education are offered for the stress of following a modified diet. Instrumental types of support, such as transportation to the grocery store or home delivered meals are offered for the stress of functional limitations. Functional status and instrumental help have a joint effect on dietary quality. In general, satisfaction with the level of all types of nutrition-related support is good in this group of women.

## DISCUSSION

This study focused on only one portion of the proposed model of social relationships and diet quality—the associations between social support, stress, and diet. The results demonstrate a joint effect of social support and functional status on diet quality. In other words, the influence of social support on diet quality varies with the level of functional status, and vice versa, the influence of functional status on diet quality varies with the level of social support.

Furthermore, interpretation of the first order effects shows that the conditional effect of functional status at the mean level of social support (1.3 helpers) is nonsignificant. That is, when the level of help is approximately one person, the predicted diet quality of all subjects is roughly equivalent. The difference in diet quality attributable to functional status occurs at higher levels of help. The conditional effect of social support at the mean level of functional disability (moderately disabled) is statistically significant.

Stated succinctly, a diet of better than average quality is associated with receiving help from more than one person for women who are not severely disabled. A diet of less than average quality is associated with receiving no help or being severely disabled.

The women were asked if they feel that the amount of help they receive is sufficient. For women receiving help, no difference in the number of providers exists between those who feel they would like more help (n=12) and those who felt the present level of help is sufficient (n=65) (t=-0.89, ns). The 12 dissatisfied women may perceive insufficient quality rather than quantity of support. Unfortunately, only eight of the 22 women who do not receive help were asked if they feel they could use some aid with food acquisition. Only one woman stated she would like *"a little more help."* She had no functional impairments.

However, some of these women appear to be in a precarious situation, especially women who receive help from one informal source only. For instance, the sole helper of one subject recently experienced a major health crisis. The helper is recovering at her daughter's house in Texas and her return to CT is uncertain. Another subject receives help from her daughter who recently purchased a second home in Florida. The subject expressed concern about her ability to procure foods in the coming winter. Loss of a "high helper" could affect many individuals. "High helpers" are fellow residents that supply significant amounts of aid to their neighbors.

Thus, qualitative and quantitative indicators suggest that food acquisition support is insufficient for some of these women. Misguided support is also evident. Misguided support, or oversupport, discussed briefly in Chapter 3, exists when the provider and recipient of support hold different interpretations of the situation. In the model of social relationships and diet quality, oversupport is a function of social integration. Rook (1985) states that the primary function of social integration is social control.

In the key informant interviews, oversupport for food acquisition was discussed by one woman. She conceded that her daughter is not allowing her to be food independent. Misguided support was reported more frequently in the areas of emotional and informational help for modified diets. The structured interviews with the larger sample revealed that 21% of the women receiving diet support perceive oversupport. Unsolicited advice was reported most frequently, followed by controlling directives, and unwanted self-disclosures.

Social isolation is another indicator of social integration. In this study, social anchorage was assessed. No correlation was found between social anchorage and dietary or demographic variables, including MAR, DQI, total calories, functional status, age, years at the complex, years alone, or rent. Although Hanson, Mattisson, and Steen (1987) found an association between BMI and social anchorage in Swedish males, no correlation exists in this sample.

Social anchorage was significantly correlated with some support measures, including general help received ($r=.32$, $p=.001$), help extended to others ($r=.34$, $p=.0005$), and diet help ($r=.24$, $p=.02$), but not with food acquisition help. After considering the items in the scale, one additional association was examined. Interestingly, social anchorage was correlated with subjective interviewer assessment of affect ($r=-.53$, $p=.0001$).

In summary, social anchorage did not demonstrate an effect on diet quality as predicted by the proposed model. However, this scale may not be an appropriate indicator of social isolation. An alternative proxy for social isolation is the absence of informal nutrition support. Women in this study who receive help from formal sources only or no help at all have diets of lower quality than women who receive help from informal sources (DQI $t=2.02$, $p=.05$; MAR $t=-1.95$, $p=.05$). Total caloric intake and BMI do not differ between these two groups.

The third dimension of social relationships proposed by the model is companionship. This study did not assess companionship nor self worth. However, one of the unexpected findings from this research is that within each functional status category (except the severely impaired) a greater number of support providers is associated with a diet of better quality. According to Rook (1985), the goal of support is to return a stressed individual to their prior level of well being. In contrast, companionship can enhance well being. Thus, in this study the effects of companionship may have been operating when both function and support were high.

## LIMITATIONS

The cross-sectional data for this study are based on self-report from a small, opportunistic sample of elderly women. The results may only be generalizable to old-old, female residents of government subsidized housing. Prior research has shown that residents of assisted housing for the elderly report larger friendship networks, smaller informal support networks, and larger formal support networks than elders living in the general community (Struyk et al. 1989). Thus, the findings, especially the descriptive results of this study, may not be applicable to community dwelling elderly. Furthermore, socially isolated women in public housing are most likely under-represented in this sample.

The use of cross-sectional data indicates that differences between groups may be influencing results. The question, *"How does diet quality change with increases in social support or with declines in functional status?"* can only be extrapolated from this cross-sectional data. A longitudinal study is necessary to assess changes over time.

In this study, individuals who are high versus low functioning, or those with high versus low levels of help may differ in other ways besides functional status or social support. For instance, the diet quality of high functioning women who receive help is better than the diet quality of high functioning women who receive no help. Perhaps an exogenous effect is influencing both acceptance of help and healthful eating habits. Thus, merely offering additional support will not change the dietary habits of current nonusers of help.

Alternative explanations exist for the differences in diet quality at various levels of functional status and social support. As noted in Chapter 7, moderated regression relies on extreme cases to detect joint effects. Subject selection and measurement error, especially in the instance of extreme cases, will influence the location of the crossover point in the regression lines and subsequent interpretation of results.

Survey data collected from older adults is particularly susceptible to certain biases. Taylor-Davis and Smiciklas-Wright (1993) report that inaccurate responses from elders are often attributable to misinterpretation of the question, motivation to answer accurately, and memory performance.

The findings from the qualitative phase were used to reduce potential sources of misinterpretation. The nutrition support questionnaire items were carefully worded in the phrases of the focus group participants and key informants. However, Taylor-Davis and Smiciklas-Wright (1993) offer the example of functional status instruments, which were also employed in this study. They report that older adults are likely to base their response on past performance and old beliefs, rather than actual recent behavior.

Memory performance is enhanced by specific prompts. The food frequency questionnaire was particularly dependent on memory; thus the interviewers used memory prods and clarified any questionable answers. For example, if the participant stated that she never drank milk, but then reported eating cereal daily, the interviewer checked for milk on the cereal.

However, motivation may have decreased accuracy. As discussed in Chapter 6, food frequencies are prone to overestimation of foods considered healthful (Salvini et al. 1989). Taylor-Davis and Smiciklas-Wright (1993) state that older adults are more likely than younger adults to report socially desirable behaviors. In other words, the tendency to under-report consumption of high fat foods and high sodium foods and to over-report consumption of fruits and vegetables would be extremely likely in this sample.

These accumulated inaccuracies are the source of measurement error. In the statistical method of moderated multiple regression, measurement error is magnified because of the product term. Measurement error combined with reliance on extreme cases decreases the likelihood of detecting joint effects.

In addition, the statistical equations being tested were likely to be nonlinear. The summary indices of diet quality have both upper and lower threshold values. Therefore, quality would be expected to taper as it approached the threshold limit. For example, consider the case of women with no physical disabilities. The improvement in diet quality between one to two helpers would be expected to be greater than the improvement from four to five helpers.

However, statistical detection of curvilinear trends is difficult, because of limitations similar to those in detection of joint effects (Pedhazur 1997). The amplification of error due to the squared term is especially problematic. Statistical detection of both joint and curvilinear effects in a nonexperimental situation is unlikely.

Lastly, this study focused on only one model of social relationships, developed from the summary of literature by Rook (1985). Her conclusions endorse a moderating effect of social support. Alternative models offer different explanations for the associations between constructs. For instance, the suppressor model is one frequently investigated, alternative model of social support, stress, and well being. Thoits (1982) and Payne and Jones (1987), among others, argue for a suppressor effect of social support.

The suppressor model is depicted below.

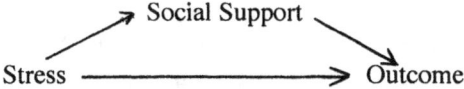

In the suppressor model, social support has a constant effect on the outcome variable (Wheaton 1985). However, the constant effect is influenced by the level of stress. Thus, social support suppresses the net effect of stress on well being. Main effects in multiple regression analysis represent suppressor effects.

The results of this study uphold the buffering model in the specific case of functional status, nutrition-related social support, and diet quality. A statistically significant joint effect indicates that the first order terms are conditional effects, not main effects, for these particular measures.

However, suppressor effects may be evident in the relationships between other measures of functional status, nutrition-related social support and diet quality. Furthermore, Wheaton (1985) posits that suppressor and buffering effects may simultaneously coexist. Thus, the current study is restrained by the limitations of variable measurement and the statistical techniques employed.

## RECOMMENDATIONS

This research has numerous limitations. The data are subjective responses. The model may be misspecified. Generalizability is limited. Nonetheless, the results do afford insights into the relationships between social support, nutrition-related stress, and diet quality. The following recommendations for policy and program design and recommendations for further research are based on careful interpretation of the findings.

## Policy and Program Implications

This study generated a wealth of descriptive and analytic results. This information should be considered when planning policies and programs designed for older adults.

### Nutrition Education

The objectives of nutrition education programs often focus on improving (changing) current eating behaviors of the learner. Stages of change theory suggests that learners must progress through a series of steps in order to implement change. The steps progress from precontemplation, to contemplation, prepreparation, action, and finally maintenance.

The results of this research indicate the current stages for these subjects as a group. For instance, osteoporosis was rarely mentioned during any focus groups or key informant interviews, and calcium intake was inadequate for many. Thus, this group of women appears to be at the precontemplation level for the problem of osteoporosis.

In contrast, reducing the intake of dietary fat was mentioned at all focus groups. Many of the key informants discussed their efforts to decrease the intake of foods high in saturated fat. The results of the food frequencies demonstrated that about half of the women are meeting current dietary recommendations. Thus, while the women appear aware of the need for dietary change, further improvement in actual intake is desirable. The stage of change is more at the level of contemplation or prepreparation.

In addition to offering nutrition education to older adults, efforts should be directed toward educating the nutrition-related support network members. The results of this research demonstrate that daughters are the most frequent source of nutrition information and advice on modified diets. At the same time, other network members are impacting food intake through their help with food acquisition. Both the informational and emotional sources of support and the instrumental sources of support must receive the nutrition education message to facilitate dietary change of elders.

Nutrition education efforts are a natural starting point for emotional and informational support of modified diets. While almost all of the subjects in this study follow dietary restrictions, perceptions of emotional and informational support were very low. Yet, these types of support could significantly improve dietary compliance. Nutrition educators are in a prominent position to offer diet instruction, reassurance, encouragement, and directives. Furthermore, nutrition educators can train other individuals, including current support providers, to offer emotional support for modified diets.

*Food Acquisition Programs*

Food acquisition is a high priority concern of this group of women. Those who are the most disabled receive the most help with this task. However, the results of this study indicate that the diet quality of women without severe disabilities is better for those who receive help than for those who do not. Thus, food acquisition programs should not be limited to elderly individuals with disabilities. Women with moderate, mild, or no disabilities may benefit from consuming a diet of high quality, thus prolonging the period of high functioning and reducing the need for additional services.

A program to encourage support for independent elders could be as simple as a community awareness campaign, or could involve recruitment of volunteers, rearranging existing services, or managing formal providers. The goal would be a low cost program to enhance access to food.

For example, milk delivery service is often associated with families having children. Yet much evidence exists that older adults, especially women, would benefit by increased consumption of low-fat dairy products. A campaign to increase the use of milk delivery by elders might prove cost effective by improving nutritional status and delaying osteoporotic fracture. A more extensive campaign could tie in delivery of additional foods, such as orange juice or fresh produce, with the milk.

Re-evaluation of the formal systems includes the bus system and congregate meals. While 75% of these women do not drive, only 13 consider public transportation a viable option to the grocery store. Congregate meals are also poorly utilized without apparent nutrition benefit. Perhaps changes could be made within these programs to improve older adults' access to food.

For many of these subjects, grocery shopping is a stressful, exhausting task. Simultaneously, grocery shopping is a major outing and social event. Of the 91 women who do their own shopping, 30 are always accompanied for health and safety reasons. Most of the women who are accompanied have moderate to severe disabilities, but 10% with mild or no disabilities are also accompanied. Some women report that they try to shop frequently to decrease anxiety and reduce fatigue. While this plan has merit, not all women have the option. A program to encourage "buddies" for brief shopping excursions might increase access to food.

The stressor examined in this study was functional status—a chronic type of stress. Even the most highly functioning women experience other types of stress, such as acute illness, mourning, or daily hassles. During these volatile periods, diet quality might be enhanced if low levels of food acquisition support are available. Thus, occasional shopping and transportation help appear important for women at all levels of function.

Furthermore, the results suggest that older adults desire to balance reciprocity. Thus, food acquisition programs would need to incorporate some method of exchange for services or sliding payment system. The Project SHARE model could work well here. Project SHARE is a cooperative food buying program. Participants qualify to purchase food packages at roughly half the retail price by completing two hours of community service each month.

Alternatively, the "exchange rate" could be more strictly defined. For instance, spending X dollars at a certain grocery store would qualify an individual for one free grocery delivery. Or a designated weight of recyclable materials could entitle an individual to a free taxicab ride. As discussed in Chapter 4, these participants stockpile food for use during a time of stress. In the same way, they would be likely to save a grocery delivery coupon for use when they catch the flu, or a taxi pass for use when the roads are icy. Program participation may be increased when older adults must "earn the right" to be enrolled.

Mor-Barak, Miller, and Syme (1991) caution that support intervention programs create social change. New sources of support must be careful to supplement, rather than supplant, current provision of support. Furthermore, stress reduction may be a preferable goal. For instance, a motorized scooter for grocery shopping may be the preferred intervention for a physically impaired, but otherwise independent elder. Provision of a homemaker aide might decrease independence and disrupt the existing support network.

*Nutrition Risk Assessment*

Primary care physicians, hospital discharge personnel, community and clinical dietitians, social service workers, and others are interested in assessing the nutritional risk of elderly clients. The Nutrition Screening Initiative has identified social isolation as one of seven key risk indicators (White 1991). Yet, for lack of a better measure, the Level 1 and Level II screens only inquire if the individual lives and eats alone (Lipschitz and White 1991).

The results of this study demonstrate that a thorough assessment of support adequacy must consider both the level of stress and the level of support. However, a quick indicator is often desirable, as in the Level I and II screens. The presence of at least one active provider of instrumental support may provide just such a measure. For instance, a simple question could be, *Is there anyone who presently picks up a few items for you at the grocery store, drives or accompanies you there, or completes your grocery shopping?* An affirmative answer would indicate a desirable situation; a negative response would indicate a precarious situation.

When at least one individual provides active help with grocery acquisition, no effect of functional status on diet quality is apparent. In addition, related research suggests that the one active support provider will help the recipient to access desired additional support (Antonucci and Akiyama 1995; Armstrong and Goldsteen 1990). For high functioning individuals, the presence of one active provider of support indicates that diet quality is enhanced in comparison to individuals with no support. Furthermore, if functional decline occurs, an initial support system will have been identified.

Increasing the complexity of the question will yield a better estimate of risk. By assessing the absolute number of helpers as 0, 1, or ≥ 2, risk can be further differentiated as high, moderate, or low, respectively. Determination of risk can be further refined by simultaneously assessing functional status.

**Further Research**

Directions for further research in the area of nutrition-related social support appear almost endless. This study focused on the interrelationship between functional status and instrumental support in women over 75 who live alone in government subsidized housing. Results are needed from similar studies with other age groups, other living situations and male gender to provide additional insight to the interrelationships between the variables. Furthermore, longitudinal studies would clarify the present findings.

Functional disability is a chronic stress, and only one of several possible nutrition-related stressors identified during the focus groups. Examination of the impact of acute stress, such as a fracture or acute illness, would further broaden our understanding of the social support process. The types, providers, and overall response rate could differ in the acute situation.

As discussed in the section on limitations, alternative models of the social support process need to be considered. The results of this research suggest two important considerations for all studies of nutrition-related social support:

 a. inclusion of nutrition-related stress, and
 b. a careful definition of social support.

Measurement of support from the viewpoint of an objective researcher might prove to have a closer relationship to diet quality. The interview with Ella illustrates the difference in the perspective of the researcher and the elderly subject. During this interview, the subject received two phone calls. Both were relatives asking Ella if she was O.K., or needed anything. Toward the end of the interview, Ella's son walked in with a bag of groceries. In spite of all this presumable support, Ella reported no instrumental or emotional help.

Other reasons could explain this particular situation. Ella may have informed her relatives about the interview. Perhaps they were worried and unusually attentive. Alternatively, Ella may have considered her relatives intrusive and unhelpful. Simultaneous evaluations of support by researchers and subjects could resolve these questions.

The perspectives of support providers would also provide increased understanding. Relationships require exchanges between individuals. The nature of these interchanges and the quality of the relationships may influence the support process.

Finally, future research needs to examine the influence of other functions of social relationships. Social integration and companionship may also impact eating behaviors. In fact, the three functions of social relationships are likely to be interrelated themselves, creating some of the conflicting results of prior research. Simultaneous consideration of all three functions would be ideal.

## CONCLUSION

In conclusion, the results of this study indicate that nutrition-related social support consists of emotional, informational, and instrumental forms of help. Like other types of social support, nutrition-related support is enacted in response to a specific stress. Elderly women who live alone in government subsidized housing are receiving instrumental support for help with grocery acquisition. The support is moderating the effect of functional status on diet quality.

Some recommendations are offered based on the results. Nutrition education efforts need to reach both the elder and the nutrition-related support providers. Food acquisition programs should be extended to women at all levels of functional ability. A simple indicator of support is the number of active providers of instrumental assistance. Finally, additional research is needed to further our understanding of nutrition-related social support.

The population of U.S. elderly is expected to double during the next half century. As the numbers increase, so will the need for social support from family, friends, and professionals. Optimal nutrition, combined with adequate support, will enhance quality of life during those later years.

# Appendices

*Appendices*  187

Appendix A: Moderator Guide

## FOCUS GROUP MODERATOR GUIDE

### INTRODUCTION

Hello, my name is Michelle Pierce.... I'm interested in what types of things influence people to eat the way they do....

First, I'd like to thank you all for volunteering to meet with me. I really appreciate your interest in this project and your time and effort to get here.

Let me tell you a little bit more about this project. The Nutrition Department at the University of Connecticut is conducting a large research study. Last year, the residents of several housing sites completed surveys asking about grocery shopping, eating out, preferred foods, etc. Perhaps some of you filled out one of these written surveys.

The next step is to talk with groups of women like yourself about food and nutrition issues. We are trying to learn what kinds of things you, and women like you, think about when trying to decide what foods to buy or what to eat at the next meal.

I am passing out a brief overview which explains that any information you tell me today will be strictly confidential. Let me read it.

You may keep the top page. If you have any questions in the future, you will have a phone number to call. Please write your name on the attached page and pass it to me now. This way we will know that you participated so that we do not invite you again in later parts of the study. Your names will not be kept with the results of today's discussion.

I am going to ask a few questions now. I want to hear what each of you has to say in response to these questions. So please, only one person talk at a time.

### QUESTIONS

(5 min)
1. For the first question only, we will go around the circle and have each person take a turn. First state your name. Then please tell us your most favorite food and your least liked food. O.K., that's name - most liked food - least liked food. We'll start with Mrs. _____ on my right and go around the circle.

(10 min)
2. For this next question, and the rest of the questions, I would like you to think of how your neighbors and friends would answer as well as yourself.

I would like you to think about your dinner meal. How do you decide what you will be eating? What kinds of things do you consider?
(Note when someone mentions "good for you", "healthful", etc. Move on to next question.)

(10 min)
3. Mrs. _____ mentioned that it should be good for you. How do you decide what is good for you?

(25 min)
4. Even though you know what foods are good for you, sometimes you can't eat the things you should. Sometimes, of course, you just feel like eating junk food, and that's O.K. But sometimes you might like to be eating better, but you can't. What are some of the problems that you might experience that make it hard to eat the foods you think you should?
(prompts: procuring, preparing, eating, digesting?)

(10 min)
5. What makes it sometimes difficult to know what is healthful and what is not?

( 5 min)
6. (List all the problems that have been discussed in large print on a big sheet of newsprint.) Can you think of any other reasons why you (or your friends or neighbors) might not be able to eat a healthful diet?

( 5 min)
7. On the top of this paper which I am now handing out, I would like you to write down the three problems which you feel are the most common among women like yourself. That is, which three do you think most people like yourself experience?
On the bottom of the paper, I would like you to write the three problems that you feel have the biggest impact on what women like yourself eat. You may write a problem on the top and bottom of the page if you think it is really common and has a big impact on food choices.
I would also appreciate it if you would write down any additional comments that you may have about any of the topics we discussed today. Perhaps we didn't have enough time for you to bring up a point, or perhaps something important occurred to you after we had moved to a new topic.

CLOSING
Would you please pass the sheets of paper to me? That was my last question. Is there anything else that any of you would like to add to the discussion, which we did not cover? Do you have any questions for me?

Appendix B: Key Informant Interview Guide

ID: _____ Date: _____
Name: _____
Address: _____

Phone: _____

**UNIVERSITY OF CONNECTICUT**
**FAMILY NUTRITION PROGRAM**


"Hello, I'm Michelle Pierce...." introduce self.

"Before we even begin, I want to thank you so much for participating in this study. First, I want to give you a brief idea of what this is all about."

Hand "Participation Consent" to interviewee. Read. (Insert ..."we aren't going to be talking too much about food per se, rather, who you discuss food issues with.") Obtain signatures on two copies. Give interviewee one copy.

### Open-ended Social Support Questionnaire

"I've been talking with a number of women like yourself, similar in age and living in an apartment building like this one. What I've come up with is a number of nutrition-related statements that many of the women have experienced. What I would like to know is which of these statements have been true for you in the last year. There are no right or wrong answers. I'm simply trying to find out how common these are."

Read each card. "Has this been true for you in the past year or not?"
Form two piles. Wrap a rubber band around the pile of concerns not experienced. Hand pile experienced to respondent.

"I would now like you to divide these into two piles. The first pile will be ones that are strongly true for you. The second pile should be those that are more minor, sometimes true and sometimes not, or simply less important to you than the issues you put in the first pile." Record letters:
MAJOR
MINOR

Lay out the cards in the MAJOR pile. "What we are most interested in for this research project is who you talk to about food or nutrition issues. So, what I would like you to do is pick out one of these that you talked about with someone else or one that somebody else helped you with. I'd like to hear all the specifics of who you talked with, how they helped, if they helped. That sort of thing. (May go on with "Again, there is no right or wrong with this. Everything that you tell me is confidential. I will never be reporting any names....")

"I would really appreciate it if I could tape record this portion of the interview. I will be taking notes also, but sometimes I miss some important points and I might want to listen again to your exact words to fill in the gaps in my notes. The tape will not be labeled with your name. Is it all right if I turn on the tape recorder?"

PROBES

a) "Specifically, who did you talk with about this?"

b) "How has X become involved in helping you deal with the problem or your feelings about it?"

c) "Is there anything in particular about X as a person or about his/her way of helping you deal with the problem that stands out for you?"

Helpers: friends or neighbors; family members; doctors, nurses, other health professionals; priest, rabbi, minister; social worker; government or housing agency worker; paid worker; volunteer?

(Probes *b* and *c* from Gottlieb 1978)

*Appendices*

Appendix C: Brief SNAP Survey

## SENIOR NUTRITION AWARENESS PROGRAM SURVEY

Please complete the following questions by placing a check in the appropriate blank.

1. Are you _____ male _____ female?

2. Do you feel that the way you eat is the best for your health?
    _____ Always
    _____ Usually
    _____ Sometimes
    _____ Never

3. Are you on a special diet? _____Yes _____ No

    Type: _____

4. How would you rate your health?
    _____ Excellent
    _____ Good
    _____ Fair
    _____ Poor

5. When were you born?
    _____ 1910 or prior
    _____ 1911 to 1920
    _____ 1921 or later

6. SNAP staff are interviewing a small number of residents. If you might possibly be available for an interview, be sure to include your name and phone number below. If you are selected, and complete the interviews, you will receive a $10.00 gratuity for your time and contribution.
    Name: _____
    Phone number: _____
    Apartment: _____Number: _____

Appendix D: Senior Eating Survey (Fey-Yensan 1995)

**SENIOR EATING SURVEY**
*Copyright 1993 Nancy Fey-Yensan*

Please help us learn more about how Seniors shop, eat and cook by completely filling out this survey. Since your name will never be used on the survey, all of your answers will be anonymous. Please take your time choosing the answers that best fit the way you shop, eat and cook, but please try not to think too hard about the questions.

Instructions: Please rank each of the statements in the survey using the scale.

| 1 | 2 | 3 | 4 | 5 |
|---|---|---|---|---|
| Never | Rarely | Sometimes | Usually | Always |

_____ I shop with a list.
_____ I eat alone.
_____ I enjoy cooking.
_____ I watch TV while eating.
_____ I look for new recipes to try.
_____ I plan my meals in advance.
_____ I use coupons when I shop for food.
_____ I prepare my meals or my family's meals.
_____ I eat breakfast.
_____ I shop for my own/my family's food.
_____ I prefer to eat alone.
_____ I am disappointed when I eat.
_____ I browse through cookbooks to plan my meals.
_____ I limit the amount of salt that I use.
_____ I buy foods that are on sale.
_____ I eat meals in restaurants with friends or relatives.
_____ I eat lunch.
_____ I enjoy sweet foods.
_____ I skip meals.
_____ I eat high fiber foods.
_____ My ability to get my groceries home can affect which foods I buy.
_____ I look forward to eating.
_____ I use canned vegetables more than fresh.

_____ I feel frustrated when I eat.
_____ I shop on a certain day of the week.
_____ I like to shop for food.
_____ Eating is a chore for me.
_____ I make baked goods for friends or relatives.
_____ I do other things while eating (reading, writing, etc.)
_____ I enjoy eating.
_____ I use canned fruits.
_____ I eat in restaurants by myself.
_____ I feel satisfied after I eat.
_____ I buy fresh foods instead of frozen or canned.
_____ I will skip a meal rather than eat alone.
_____ I have friends or relatives over to meals.
_____ I enjoy eating in other people's homes.
_____ I eat supper.
_____ I forget to eat meals.
_____ I make special foods for my guests.
_____ I feel like nothing is safe to eat anymore.
_____ I eat canned meats (chicken, pork, beef).
_____ When I'm hungry, I eat whatever's quickest.
_____ I enjoy the aroma (smell) of foods.
_____ I make brewed coffee (not instant) at home.
_____ I eat better when I eat with someone.
_____ I buy baked goods from a bakery or super-market.
_____ I use food stamps.
_____ I eat fresh fruits and vegetables.
_____ Food tastes good to me.
_____ I enjoy eating foods with different textures (smooth, crunchy, etc.)
_____ Someone else helps me shop for food.
_____ I rely on easy to prepare foods to make meals for myself.
_____ I can tell what herbs and spices are in foods.
_____ I avoid eating when I am hungry.
_____ I need help shopping for food.
_____ I take my time while eating.
_____ Eating meals is the most enjoyable part of my day.
_____ I eat differently on the weekends than during the week.
_____ I eat when it's mealtime, whether I'm hungry or not.
_____ Someone else prepares meals for me.
_____ I avoid sour tasting foods (like citrus fruits).
_____ I view cooking as just another chore.
_____ I eat more when I am worried or upset.
_____ I eat the same foods day after day.
_____ I enjoy salty foods.
_____ How a food looks will determine whether I will eat it or not.

_____ I eat frozen dinners or frozen meals (like Le Menu, TV dinners, Healthy Choice, etc.).
_____ I read cooking or food magazines or articles.
_____ I read food labels to help me make food choices at the store.
_____ I have a good appetite.
_____ I add hot pepper (black or red) to my foods.
_____ I make baked goods from boxed mixes.
_____ I like to cook for myself.
_____ I use herbs and spices in place of salt.
_____ I like to spend time preparing meals.
_____ I enjoy having guests over for meals.
_____ I add salt to my food before I taste it.
_____ When I overeat, I feel guilty.
_____ I eat canned entrees at home (chili, beef stew, spaghetti, etc.)
_____ I decide what foods are served in my home.
_____ I make homemade soups.
_____ I eat low-fat foods.
_____ I need help preparing meals.
_____ Food is an important part of my life.
_____ I snack between meals or in the evening (include waking up in the middle of the night to get something to eat).
_____ I limit the amount of fat and cholesterol in my diet.
_____ I nibble while meals are being prepared.
_____ I have enough money to buy all of the foods I need.
_____ I make baked goods from scratch.
_____ I eat canned soups.
_____ I try newly advertised food products.
_____ I overeat.
_____ I will skip meals if what I like is not available.
_____ Spending money in a restaurant is a waste for me.
_____ I use frozen vegetables.
_____ I enjoy eating with other people.
_____ I use canned fish (tuna, sardines, salmon) or frozen fish products more than fresh fish.

*Used with permission of the author.*

Appendix E: Nutrition Social Support Questionnaire

## Social Support Information Sheet

ID # _____
Date _____
Interviewer _____

*Introduce self.*
Some of today's questions are similar to questions asked in the previous interviews. We wanted more detail on some of the issues and that is why I will be asking them again.

I am first going to ask some questions about people that you help and people who help you. We are going to talk about people who are important to you, so I have found that using first names is easiest.

Let me just add here also that all of the information that you tell me is strictly confidential. The information that you give me will not be paired with your name on any of our records.

O.K. to start?

1. People sometimes help each other by giving advice, assistance, or moral support. Is there anyone who turns to you for these kinds of help?

_____ No ---> *Go to next question.*
Yes ---> Specifically, who looks to you for help? Please give me their first name.

First Name
_____
_____
_____
_____
_____
_____

*Prompts:* Family Members: daughters, sons, sisters, brothers, in-laws, grandchildren
Health Care Workers: doctors, nurses, VNA, aides, companions, dieticians, friendly visitor
Friends or Neighbors
Housing Staff: site manager, social worker, service coordinator

1A. Total # from 1 (above): _____

2. When you need help, like advice, assistance, or moral support, is there anyone that you turn to?

_____ No ---> *Go to next question.*
_____ Yes ---> Specifically, who do you look to for help? Please give me their first name.

First Name

_____
_____
_____
_____
_____
_____
_____
_____

*Prompts:* Family Members: daughters, sons, sisters, brothers, in-laws, grandchildren,
Health Care Workers: doctors, nurses, VNA, aides, companions, dieticians, friendly visitor
Friends or Neighbors
Housing Staff: site manager, social worker, service coordinator

2A. Total # from 2 (above): _____

# Appendices

Now I am going to ask you some questions about any special diet that you may follow and about the people that might help you with this.

3. Has a physician ever told you to follow a special diet?

_____ No = 0 --> *Go to question #6B.*
Yes --> What type? *(Circle all that apply.)*

1) Diabetic (exchange plan)
2) Lactose free
3) Low cholesterol
4) Low fat
5) Low fiber
6) Low sodium
7) Low sugar
8) Low starch
9) Weight gain
10) Weight loss *(If only "10", skip to question #6B.)*
11) Other: _____
12) High complex carbohydrate
13) More fruits and vegetables
14) More calcium
15) High fiber
16) Avoid foods that don't agree (ex. heartburn, diverticulitis/osis)

Did your doctor have any other recommendations?

4. *(If "10",* Excluding weight reduction, weight loss is addressed in a later question) During the past year, would you say that you followed the doctor's recommendations

1) Almost always
2) Often
3) Sometimes
4) Seldom
5) Almost never

5. How important is following the doctor's recommendations to you?

1) Very important
2) Somewhat important
3) Relatively unimportant

*If yes doctor diet:*
6A. In addition to what your doctor prescribed, is there anything else that you try to watch when you eat?

*If no doctor diet:*
6B. Is there anything that you try to watch when you eat?

_____ No = 0 --> *Go to question #9.*
Yes --> Specifically, what do you try to watch?
*(Circle all that apply.)*
*(Open ended, no prompts.)*

1) Diabetic (exchange plan)
2) Lactose free
3) Low cholesterol
4) Low fat
5) Low fiber
6) Low sodium
7) Low sugar
8) Low starch
9) Weight gain
10) Weight loss *(If only "10", skip to question #9.)*
11) Other: _____

12) High complex carbohydrate
13) More fruits and vegetables
14) More calcium
15) High fiber
16) Avoid foods that don't agree (ex. heartburn, diverticulitis/osis)

Anything else?

7. (*If "10"*, Excluding weight reduction, weight loss is addressed in a later question) Thinking of just this past year, would you say that when you ate you considered _____ *(items mentioned above,)*

1) Almost always
2) Often
3) Sometimes
4) Seldom
5) Almost never

8. How important is eating this way to you?

1) Very important
2) Somewhat important
3) Relatively unimportant

# Appendices

9. During the past year, have you tried to lose weight?

　　____No = 0 ---> *Go to question #11.*
　　　　Yes --> Just in the last year, would you say that you followed a reducing diet or tried to limit the amount of food that you ate

　　　　　　1) Almost always　　　4) Seldom
　　　　　　2) Often　　　　　　　5) Almost Never
　　　　　　3) Sometimes

10. How important is losing weight to you?

　　　　1) Very important　　2) Somewhat important　　3) Relatively unimportant

*Interviewer Note: For numbers 11 and 12 below, only document net weight loss, not any pounds lost and subsequently regained.*

11. In the past year, have you lost any weight? _____ # pounds net loss

12. In the past 5 years, have you lost any weight? _____ # pounds net loss

13. *Mark here with "N" if No --->* _____ *#3,* _____ *#6,* _____ *#9. If all three = No, then say "I am going to skip ahead here. These questions do not apply since you do not follow a special diet". Go to* **********************.
No special diet code = 9 (N/A).　　　　　　　*(If #3, #6, or #9 = yes, continue.)*

　　We are very interested in learning who helps older adults follow special diets or healthful ways of eating. In interviewing other older women, I have learned that people have helped them in a number of ways. People have helped by giving information about foods; or by offering suggestions or advice. People have provided encouragement. People have helped by sharing how they handle a similar healthful diet. In other instances, women that I have interviewed have received no help in following their diet or in trying to eat healthfully.
　　I would like you to think back over the **past year, just in the past year,** and tell me if there is anyone who has helped you to follow your special diet or to eat in a more healthful way.

　　　　No --> *See prompts.*
　　____Still No = 0, *Go to question #14.*
　　____Yes = 1 --> *Go to question #15.*

*Prompts:* Family Members: daughters, sons, sisters, brothers, in-laws, grandchildren,
Health Care Workers: doctors, nurses, VNA, aides, companions, dieticians, friendly visitor
Friends or Neighbors
Housing Staff: site manager, social worker, service coordinator

14. **Do you feel that if you had some support you would be better able to** follow your diet / eat the way you feel you should, **or do you feel that you are quite capable on your own?**

_____A. Capable on own = 0 ---> *Go to question 18.*
       Would like support = 1 ---> *For each of the following, please indicate if you would like this type of aid or not.*

$$\text{No} = 0, \text{Yes} = 1, \text{N/A} = 9$$

  B. Suggestions or advice regarding the way you should eat
  C. Reassurance or encouragement to eat the way you should
  D. Information or education about the way you should eat
  E. Talking with others who follow a similar diet
  F. Firm directions on what you should or shouldn't eat
  G. Other: _____

*Go to question 18.*

15. Please tell me the first name or names of the people who have helped you.

  As I mentioned, in my previous interviews I have noticed a number of ways that people help each other. I would like to know if the individual(s) that you mentioned has helped you in any of these ways.
  *(Hold chart.)* I have a list here of ways of helping. There are certainly many other ways of helping, but these are the ones I've seen most frequently when I talk to people about diet. *(Hand chart.)* Sometimes helpers ... *(read chart).*
  I am now going to read statements corresponding to these ways of helping. (Don't answer this right now but) for instance, "Does _____ offer suggestions or advice that help you to eat healthfully?". Simply answer "yes" if this is true, or "no" if it is not. You may answer as many "yes's" or "no's" as you want. There is no right or wrong way to answer. It is simply how you feel about the people you mentioned.

Appendices

**A. Does _____ help you to** follow your diet / eat healthier? (No => Anyone else? *Go to prompts.*)

**1. Does _____ offer suggestions and advice that help you to** follow your diet / eat healthier?
**2. Does _____ reassure you when you do the right things to** follow your diet / eat healthier?
**3. Does _____ provide you with information or education which helps you to** better understand your diet / eat healthier?
**4. Do you talk with _____ about the way s/he eats which is somewhat similar to you, sharing feelings or the way you do things?**
**5. Does _____ tell you what to eat and not eat which helps you to** follow your diet / eat healthier?
**6. Is there anything else that _____ does that helps you to** follow your diet / eat healthier? *(Write in block below.)*

*(Interviewer Note: Be sure to type Y or N(-) in each box below.)*

| Person | 1<br>sugg/adv | 2<br>reassure | 3<br>info/edu | 4<br>same diet | 5<br>tells me | 6<br>other |
|---|---|---|---|---|---|---|
| | | | | | | |
| | | | | | | |
| | | | | | | |
| | | | | | | |
| | | | | | | |
| | | | | | | |
| | | | | | | |
| | | | | | | |

Is there anyone else that you think has helped you to follow your diet in the past year? *(Give pauses between prompts.)*

15A. Total number from 15 (above) = _____

*Prompts:* Family Members: daughters, sons, sisters, brothers, in-laws, grandchildren,
Health Care Workers: doctors, nurses, VNA, aides, companions, dieticians, friendly visitor
Friends or Neighbors
Housing Staff: site manager, social worker, service coordinator

16. Overall, would you say that you have received adequate support toward eating a healthful diet, or would you prefer more support?

_____ A. Adequate = 0 ---> *Go to next question.*
Would like more support = 1 ---> For each of the following, please indicate if you would like more of this type of aid or not. Would you like more *(Circle all that apply.)*

$$No = 0, Yes = 1, N/A = 9$$

  B. Suggestions or advice
  C. Reassurance or encouragement
  D. Information or education
  E. Talking with others who follow a similar diet
  F. Firm directions on what you should eat or shouldn't eat
  G. Other: _____

17. Do you feel that some people offer too much support; that is, you'd like a little help toward eating a healthful diet, but some people seem to go overboard?

_____ A. No = 0 ---> *Go to next question.*
Yes = 1 ---> For each of the following, please indicate if you would like less or not. Would you like less *(Circle all that apply.)*

$$No = 0, Yes = 1, N/A = 9$$

  B. Suggestions or advice
  C. Reassurance or encouragement
  D. Information or education
  E. Talking with others who follow a similar diet
  F. Firm directions on what you should eat or shouldn't eat
  G. Other: _____

# Appendices

18. Sometimes people try to help, but the assistance they offer seems either misguided or not generally useful. Can you think of anyone who tried to offer help, but you just didn't find it helpful?

\_\_\_\_\_ No --> *Go to next question.*
Yes -->Who? Specifically, what type of help did they offer?

    1) Suggestions or advice
    2) Reassurance or encouragement
    3) Information or education
    4) Talking with others who follow a similar diet
    5) Firm directions on what you should eat or shouldn't eat
    6) Other: write in block below

| Person | 1 sugg/adv | 2 reassure | 3 info/edu | 4 same diet | 5 tells me | 6 other |
|---|---|---|---|---|---|---|
| | | | | | | |
| | | | | | | |
| | | | | | | |
| | | | | | | |
| | | | | | | |
| | | | | | | |
| | | | | | | |

18A. Total # from 18 (above) = _____

19. We've been talking about the past year. Now I'd like you to think back before that. Excluding the people who are now helping you, was there anyone else who helped you in the past - help that you're not actively receiving now but that you feel is still having a positive impact on the way you eat?

_____ No --> *Go to next question.*
_____ Yes -->Who? Specifically, what type of help did they offer?

   1) Suggestions or advice
   2) Reassurance or encouragement
   3) Information or education
   4) Talking with others who follow a similar diet
   5) Firm directions on what you should eat or shouldn't eat
   6) Other: write in block below

| Year | Person | 1 sugg/ adv | 2 reassure | 3 info/edu | 4 same diet | 5 tells me | 6 other |
|------|--------|-------------|------------|------------|-------------|------------|---------|
|      |        |             |            |            |             |            |         |
|      |        |             |            |            |             |            |         |
|      |        |             |            |            |             |            |         |
|      |        |             |            |            |             |            |         |
|      |        |             |            |            |             |            |         |
|      |        |             |            |            |             |            |         |

Prompts: classes, friends, sisters, brothers, children, doctor, nurse...?

19A. Total # from 19 above = _____

*********************************************************************

The next part of the questionnaire is about people who might help you get to the grocery store, or help you with your shopping, food preparation, or cooking. We are very interested in learning if any individuals or agency programs ever help you to obtain the food that you need. Please answer the questions for the help you have received just in the past year only.

*(Interviewer note: If help received during an acute situation, record answers and note "A" and period of help.)*

*Appendices*

*Interviewer Note: Fill in the table below with the frequency of help, i.e. 2x/wk, 3x/mo, 1x/yr. (Code every other day as 3x/wk, every other week as 2x/mo.) Remember "A"=acute & time.*

20. Who does the majority of your grocery shopping? How often? *(Fill in slot under #21 if refers to small pick-ups.)* Does anyone else ever do a major trip for you? How often?

21. If you run out of items, like juice or bread, between the big shopping trips, does anyone ever pick up a these few things for you?

    \_\_\_\_\_No
        Yes --> Who picks up a few things for you? How often?
        Anyone else? How often?

22. *(If respondent does own shopping--->)* How do you get to the grocery store? Any other ways? *(Prompts: public bus, Sr. Van, walk, taxi, own car, other car,...)*

23. Does anyone ever accompany you to the grocery store for health or safety reasons, or to help you with your shopping?

    \_\_\_\_\_No
        Yes-->Who helps you? How often? Anyone else? How often?

| HELPER | HOW OFTEN? | | | |
|---|---|---|---|---|
| First name or specific transportation | 20 major shop | 21 minor shop | 22 transportation | 23 accompany |
|  |  |  |  |  |
|  |  |  |  |  |
|  |  |  |  |  |
|  |  |  |  |  |
|  |  |  |  |  |
|  |  |  |  |  |

23A. Total number of <u>people</u> from 20-23 (above) <u>excluding self</u> = _____

*Prompts:* Transportation Services: Sr. bus, public bus, taxi,     Shopping Service:
Family Members: daughters, sons, sisters, brothers, in-laws, grandchildren
Health Care Workers: doctors, nurses, VNA, aides, companions, dieticians, friendly visitor
Friends or Neighbors
Housing Staff: site manager, social worker, service coordinator

24. Overall, how satisfied are you with the amount of help that you receive in obtaining the foods that you need? Do you feel that you need
*(Interviewer Note: amount of help may equal "none".)*

    1) Much less help
    2) A little less help
    3) Satisfied with the amount of help
    4) A little more help
    5) Much more help

25. Do you take part in any meal programs, such as a lunch program, or Sr. Center meals/ church meals/ congregate meals, or breakfasts, or Meals-on-Wheels? How often?

\_\_\_\_\_ No = 0
       Yes ---> Which program(s)?

| Program | How often? |
|---------|------------|
|         |            |
|         |            |
|         |            |

Any others?

    1) congregate meals in housing site
    2) congregate meals in Sr. Center, church, other location
    3) meals-on-wheels
    4) breakfast program
    5) regularly scheduled dinners (church, Sr. Center, other)
    6) other: _____

NOTE: FOR CODING, HOW OFTEN? = NUMBER TIMES PER YEAR

*Appendices* *207*

*Interviewer Note: Fill in the table below with the frequency of help, i.e. 2x/wk, 3x/mo, 1x/yr. (Code every other day as 3x/wk, every other week as 2x/mo.) Remember, if help received during an acute situation, record answers and note "A" and period of help.)*

26. Does anyone ever help you partially prepare your food, for instance by packaging your meat in individual portions, or by cutting your vegetables before storing them in your refrigerator?

\_\_\_\_\_No
Yes---> Who helps you? How often? Anyone else? How often?

27. Does anyone bring you prepared food on a regular basis?

\_\_\_\_\_No
Yes---> Who? How often? Anyone else? How often?

28. Do you eat at anyone else's home on a regular basis?

\_\_\_\_\_No
Yes ---> Whose? How often? Anyone else? How often?

| HELPER | HOW OFTEN? | | |
|---|---|---|---|
| First name | 26 partial prep | 27 bring food | 28 eat at |
|  |  |  |  |
|  |  |  |  |
|  |  |  |  |
|  |  |  |  |
|  |  |  |  |
|  |  |  |  |

28A. Total number from 26-28 (above) = _____

*Prompts:* Family Members: daughters, sons, sisters, brothers, in-laws, grandchildren
Health Care Workers: doctors, nurses, VNA, aides, companions, dieticians, friendly visitor
Friends or neighbors
Housing Staff: site manager, social worker, service coordinator

29. Overall, how satisfied are you with the amount of help that you receive in preparing meals or in having meals provided for you? Do you feel that you need *(Interviewer Note: amount of help may equal "none".)*

       1) Much less help
       2) A little less help
       3) Satisfied with the amount of help
       4) A little more help
       5) Much more help

30. I would like a little more information about each of the people you've mentioned as helpers. Let me write their names here. *(Include all persons previously mentioned.)*

**Network Diagram**

| Helper | Relationship | How long known | Where live | | Willingness to help * |
| | | | Town (state) | Distance in time | |
|---|---|---|---|---|---|
| | | | | | |
| | | | | | |
| | | | | | |
| | | | | | |
| | | | | | |
| | | | | | |
| | | | | | |
| | | | | | |
| | | | | | |
| | | | | | |
| | | | | | |
| | | | | | |

\* Do you feel that _____ is

       1) always willing to help
       2) usually willing to help
       3) sometimes willing to help
       4) seldom willing to help
       5) rarely willing to help

*30 continued...*

**Network Diagram**

| Helper | Relationship | How long known | Where live | | Willingness to help * |
| | | | Town (state) | Distance in time | |
|---|---|---|---|---|---|
| | | | | | |
| | | | | | |
| | | | | | |
| | | | | | |
| | | | | | |
| | | | | | |
| | | | | | |
| | | | | | |
| | | | | | |
| | | | | | |
| | | | | | |
| | | | | | |
| | | | | | |
| | | | | | |
| | | | | | |
| | | | | | |
| | | | | | |
| | | | | | |

* Do you feel that _____ is

    1) always willing to help
    2) usually willing to help
    3) sometimes willing to help
    4) seldom willing to help
    5) rarely willing to help

## Ways of Helping

- Offers suggestions or advice
- Reassures or encourages
- Provides information or education
- Talks about somewhat similar diet she/he follows
- Tells you what to eat and not eat
- Other

# References

Abel, E.K. 1989. The ambiguities of social support: Adult daughters caring for frail elderly parents. *J Aging Studies* 3:211–30.

Abernathy, R.P. 1991. Body mass index: Determination and use. *J Am Diet Assoc* 91:843.

Administration on Aging. 1983. *An evaluation of the nutrition services for the elderly*. Washington, DC: DHHS.

Administration on Aging. 1994. *Report on food and nutrition for life: Malnutrition and older Americans*. Washington, DC: DHHS.

Ahmed, F.E. 1992. Effect of nutrition on the health of the elderly. *J Am Diet Assoc* 92:1102–08.

Aiken, L.S., and S.G. West. 1991. *Multiple regression: Testing and interpreting interactions*. Thousand Oaks, CA: Sage.

Antonucci, T.C. 1985. Personal characteristics, social support and social behavior. In *Handbook of aging and the social sciences*. 2$^{nd}$ ed., Ed. R.H. Binstock, and E. Shanas. New York: Van Nostrand Reinhold.

Antonucci, T.C., and H. Akiyama. 1995. Convoys of social relations: Family and friendships within a life span context. In *Handbook of aging and the family*, Ed. R. Blieszner, and V.H. Bedford. Westport, CT: Greenwood Press.

Armstrong, M.J., and K.S. Goldsteen. 1990. Friendship support patterns of older American women. *J Aging Studies* 4:391–404.

Barrera, M. 1986. Distinctions between social support concepts, measures and models. *Am J Comm Psychol* 14:413–45.

Barrera, M., I.N. Sandler, and T.B. Ramsay. 1981. Preliminary development of a scale of social support: Studies on college students. *Am J Comm Psych* 9:435–47.

Betts, N.M., and V.M. Vivian. 1985. Factors related to the dietary adequacy of noninstitutionalized elderly. *J Nutr Eld* 4:3–14.

Bianchetti, A., R. Rozzini, C. Carabellese, O. Zaneiit, and M. Trabucchi. 1990. Nutritional intake, socioeconomic conditions and health status in a large elderly population. *J Am Geri Soc* 38:521–26.

Bidlack, W.R., and W. Wang. 1995. Nutrition requirements of the elderly. In *Geriatric nutrition*. $2^{nd}$ ed., Ed. J.E. Morley, Z. Glick, and L.Z. Rubenstein. New York: Raven Press.

Biegel, D.E., K.J. Farkas, and N. Wadsworth. 1994. Social service programs for older adults and their families: Service use and barriers. In *Services to the aging and aged: Public policies and programs*, Ed. P.K.H. Kim. New York: Garland.

Blalock, H.M. 1979. *Social statistics*. $2^{nd}$ ed. New York: McGraw-Hill.

Block, G., and A.M. Hartman. 1989. Issues in reproducibility and validity of dietary studies. *Am J Clin Nutr* 50:1133–38.

Block, G., and A.F. Subar. 1992. Estimates of nutrient intake from a food frequency questionnaire: The 1987 National Health Interview Survey. *J Am Diet Assoc* 92:969–77.

Block, G., C.M. Dresser, A.M. Hartman, and M.D. Carroll. 1985. Nutrient sources in the American diet: Quantitative data from the NHANES II survey. *Am J Epidem* 122:27–40.

Block, G., A.M. Hartman, C.M. Dresser, M.D. Carroll, J. Gannon, and L. Gardner. 1986. A data-based approach to diet questionnaire design and testing. *Am J Epidem* 124:453–69.

Block, G., F.E. Thompson, A.M. Hartman, F.A. Larkin, and K.E. Guire. 1992. Comparison of two dietary questionnaires validated against multiple dietary records collected during a 1–year period. *J Am Diet Assoc* 92:686–93.

Block, G., M. Woods, A. Potosky, and C. Clifford. 1990. Validation of a self-administered diet history questionnaire using multiple diet records. *J Clin Epidem* 43:1327–35.

Bloom, J.R. 1990. The relationship of social support and health. *Soc Sci Med* 30:635–37.

BMDP Statistical Software, Inc., 1990. Statistical software version 1990. Los Angeles, CA.

Broadhead, W.E., B.H. Kaplan, S.A. James, E.H. Wagner, V.J. Schoenbach, R. Grimson, S. Heyden, G. Tibblin, and S.H. Gehlbach. 1983. The epidemiologic evidence for a relationship between social support and health. *J Epidem* 117:521–36.

Campbell, W.W., and W.J. Evans. 1996. Protein requirements of elderly people. *Euro J Clin Nutr* 50:S180–85.

Campbell, W.W., M.C. Crim, G.E. Dallal, V.R. Young, and W.J. Evans. 1994. Increased protein requirements in elderly people: New data and retrospective reassessments. *Am J Clin Nutr* 60:501–09.

Chappell, N.L., and M. Badger. 1989. Social isolation and well being. *J Geront* 44:S169–76.

Chappell, N.L., and L.W. Guse. 1989. Linkages between informal and formal support. In *Aging, stress and health*, Ed. K.S. Markides, and C.L. Cooper. New York: John Wiley & Sons.

Chiriboga, D.A. 1989. The measurement of stress exposure in later life. In *Aging, stress and health*, Ed. K.S. Markides, and C.L. Cooper. New York: John Wiley & Sons.

Clancy, K.L. 1975. Preliminary observations on media use and food habits of the elderly. *Gerontol* 15:529–32.

Coe, R.M., and D.K. Miller. 1984. Sociologic factors that influence nutritional status in the elderly. In *Nutritional intervention in the aging process*, Ed. H.J. Armbrecht, J.M. Prendergast, and R.M. Coe. New York: Springer-Verlag.

Coe, R.M., F.D. Wolinsky, D.K. Miller, and J.M. Prendergast. 1984. Complementary and compensatory functions in social network relationships among the elderly. *Gerontol* 24:396–400.

Cohen, N.L., and P.A. Ralston. 1992. *Factors influencing dietary quality of elderly blacks*. Report submitted to AARP Andrus Foundation.

Cohen, S., and T.A. Wills. 1985. Stress, social support and the buffering hypothesis. *Psych Bull* 98:310–57.

Connecticut Department on Aging. 1992. A housing directory for older adults. Hartford, CT. Photocopy.

Coulston, A.M., L. Craig, and A.C. Voss. 1996. Meals-on-wheels applicants are a population at risk for poor nutritional status. *J Am Diet Assoc* 96:570–73.

Crimmins, E.M., and Y. Saito. 1993. Getting better and getting worse: Transitions in functional status among older Americans. *J Aging Health* 5:3–36.

Crohan, S.E., and T.C. Antonucci. 1989. Friends as a source of social support in old age. In *Older adult friendship: Structure and process*, Ed. R.G. Adams, and R. Blieszner. Newbury Park, CA: Sage.

Cummings, S.R., G. Block, K. McHenry, and R.B. Baron. 1987. Evaluation of two food frequency methods of measuring dietary calcium intake. *Am J Epidem* 126:796–802.

Cutler, J.A., D. Follmann, and P.S. Allender. 1997. Randomized trials of sodium reduction: An overview. *Am J Clin Nutr* 65:643S-51.

Cutrona, C.E. 1986. Objective determinants of perceived social support. *J Person Soc Psych* 50:349–55.

Dakof, G.A., and S.E. Taylor. 1990. Victims' perceptions of social support: What is helpful from whom? *J Pers Soc Psych* 58:80–89.

Davies, L., and K.C. Knutson. 1991. Warning signals for malnutrition in the elderly. *J Am Diet Assoc* 91:1413–17.

Davis, M.A., S.P. Murphy, J.M. Neuhaus, and D. Lein. 1990. Living arrangements and dietary quality of older U.S. adults. *J Am Diet Assoc* 90:1667–72.

Davis, M.A., E. Randall, R.N. Forthofer, E.S. Lee, and S. Margen. 1985. Living arrangements and dietary patterns of older adults in the United States. *J Gerontol* 40:434–42.

Dawson-Hughes, B. 1997. Significance of habitual calcium and vitamin D intakes to post-menopausal risk of osteoporosis. Paper presented at 16$^{th}$ International Conference of Nutrition, Montreal, Canada.

de Castro, J.M. 1994. Social facilitation of food intake: People eat more with other people. *Food Nutr News* 66:29–30.

Dean, A.G., J.A. Dean, D. Coulombier, K.A. Brendel, D.C. Smith, A.H. Burton, R.C. Dicker, K. Sullivan, R.F. Fagan, R.G. Arner. 1994. Epi Info, Version 6: A word processing, database and statistics program for epidemiology on microcomputers. CDC, Atlanta, GA.

Duffy, V.B. 1993. Olfactory dysfunction, food behaviors, dietary intake and anthropometric measures in single-living, elderly women. Ph.D. diss., University of Connecticut.

Dunlap, W.P., and E.R. Kemery. 1988. Effects of predictor intercorrelations and reliabilities on moderated multiple regression. *Org Beh Hum Decision Proc* 41:248–58.

Dwyer, J.T. 1991. *Screening older Americans' nutritional health: Current practices and future possibilities*. Washington DC: Nutrition Screening Initiative.

Dwyer, J.W. 1995. The effects of illness on the family. In *Handbook of aging and the family,* Ed. R. Blieszner, and V.H. Bedford. Westport CT: Greenwood Press.

Ely, D.L. 1997. Overview of dietary sodium effects on and interactions with cardiovascular and neuroendocrine functions. *Am J Clin Nutr* 65:594S-605.

Ernst, N.D., E. Obarzanek, M.B. Clark, R.R. Briefel, C.D. Brown, and K. Donato. 1997. Cardiovascular health risks related to overweight. *J Am Diet Assoc* 97:S47–51.

Falk, L.W., C.A. Bisogni, and J. Sobal. 1996. Food choice processes of older adults: A qualitative investigation. *J Nutr Edu* 28:257–65.

Fanelli, M.T., and K.J. Stevenhagen. 1985. Characterizing consumption patterns by food frequency methods: Core foods and variety of foods in diets of older Americans. *J Am Diet Assoc* 85:1570–76.

Fey-Yensan, N. 1995. Documenting food behavior in independent-living older adults: Development and validation of a self-administered instrument. Ph.D. diss., University of Connecticut.

Fillenbaum, G.G. 1986. *Multidimensional functional assessment of older adults: The Duke older Americans resources and services procedures*. New Jersey: Lawrence Erlbaum.

Finney, J.W., R.E. Mitchell, R.C. Cronkite, and R.H. Moos. 1984. Methodological issues in estimating main and interactive effects: Examples from coping/ social support and stress field. *J Health Soc Beh* 25:85–98.

Fischer, J., and M.A. Johnson. 1990. Low body weight and weight loss in the aged. *J Am Diet Assoc* 90:1697–706.

Fitti, J., and M.G. Kovar. 1992. The longitudinal study of aging: 1984–90. *Vital and health statistics* 1(28).

Fogler-Levitt, E., D. Lau, A. Csima, M. Krondl, and P. Coleman. 1995. Utilization of home-delivered meals by recipients 75 years of age or older. *J Am Diet Assoc* 95:552–57.

Food and Nutrition Board (FNB), National Research Council. 1989. *Recommended dietary allowances*. 10th ed. Washington, DC: National Academy Press.

Frongillo, E.A., B.S. Rauschenbach, D.A. Roe, and D.F. Williamson. 1992. Characteristics related to elderly persons' not eating for 1 or more days: Implications for meal programs. *Am J Pub Health* 82:600–02.

Fulton, J.P., S. Katz, S.S. Jack, and G.H. Hendershot. 1989. Physical functioning of the aged: United States 1984. *Vital and health statistics* 10(167).

Galanos, A.N., C.F. Pieper, J.C. Cornoni-Huntley, C.W. Bales, and G.G. Fillenbaum. 1994. Nutrition and function: Is there a relationship between body mass index and the functional capabilities of community-dwelling elderly? *J Am Geri Soc* 42:368–73.

George, L.K. 1989. Stress, social support and depression over the life-course. In *Aging, stress and health,* Ed. K.S. Markides, and C.L. Cooper, New York: John Wiley and Sons.

Gibson, R.S. 1990. *Principles of nutritional assessment.* New York: Oxford.

Golant, S.M. 1992. *Housing America's elderly: Many possibilities/few choices.* Newbury Park, CA: Sage.

Gottlieb, B.H. 1978. The development and application of a classification scheme of informal helping behaviors. *Can J Beh Sci* 10:105–15.

Gray-Donald, K. 1995. The frail elderly: Meeting the nutritional challenges. *J Am Diet Assoc* 95:538–40.

Greenbaum, T.L. 1988. *The practical handbook and guide to focus group research.* Lexington, MA: Lexington Books.

Grundy, E., A. Bowling, and M. Farquhar. 1996. Social support, life satisfaction and survival at older ages. In *Health and mortality among elderly populations,* Ed. G. Caselli, and A.D. Lopez. Oxford: Clarendon Press.

Guigoz, Y. 1995. Recommended dietary allowances (RDA) for the elderly. In *Nutritional intervention and the elderly,* Ed. B.J. Vellas, P. Sachet, and R.J. Baumgartner. New York: Springer.

Guthrie, H.A., and J.C. Scheer. 1981. Validity of a dietary score for assessing nutrient adequacy. *J Am Diet Assoc* 78:240–45.

Haboubi, N.Y., P.R. Hudson, and M.S. Pathy. 1990. Measurement of height in the elderly. *J Am Geri Soc* 38:1008–10.

Ham, R.J. 1991. *Indicators of poor nutritional status in older Americans.* Washington, DC: Nutrition Screening Initiative.

Hanson, B.S., and P.O. Ostergren. 1987. Different social network and social support characteristics, nervous problems and insomnia: Theoretical and methodological aspects on some results from the population study "Men born in 1914", Malmo, Sweden. *Soc Sci Med* 25:849–59.

Hanson, B.S., I. Mattisson, and B. Steen. 1987. Dietary intake and psychosocial factors in 68–year-old men: A population study. *Compr Gerontol B* 31:53–56.

Hansson, R.O., and B.N. Carpenter. 1994. *Relationships in old age: Coping with the challenge of transition.* New York: Guilford Press.

Harris, T., M.G. Kovar, R. Suzman, J.C. Kleinman, and J.J. Feldman. 1989. Longitudinal study of physical ability in the oldest-old. *Am J Pub Health* 79:698–70.

Harrison, G.G. 1997. Reducing dietary fat: Putting theory into practice – Conference summary. *J Am Diet Assoc* 97:S93–96.

Heller, K., and W.E. Mansbach. 1984. The multifaceted nature of social support in a community sample of elderly women. *J Soc Issues* 40:99–112.

Hellman, E.A., and C. Stewart. 1994. Social support and the elderly client. *Home Health Nurs* 12:51–60.

Hendricks, J., and T.M. Calasanti. 1986. Social-psychological aspects of nutrition among the elderly Part I: Social dimensions of nutrition. In *Nutritional aspects of aging*. Vol. I. Ed. L.H. Chen. Boca Raton: CRC Press.

Hendricks, J., T.M. Calasanti, and H.B. Turner. 1988. Foodways of the elderly: Social research considerations. *Am Beh Scientist* 32:61–83.

Hinrichsen, G.A. 1985. The impact of age-concentrated, publicly assisted housing on older people's social and emotional well being. *J Gerontol* 40:758–60.

Hogan, D.P., and D.J. Eggebeen. 1995. Sources of emergency help and routine assistance in old age. *Soc Forces* 73:917–36.

Holcomb, C.A. 1995. Positive influence of age and education on food consumption and nutrient intakes of older women living alone. *J Am Diet Assoc* 95:1381–86.

Horwath, C.C. 1989. Dietary intake studies in elderly people. *World Rev Nutr Diet* 59:1–70.

Howarth, G. 1993. Food consumption, social roles and personal identity. In *Aging, independence and the life course*, Ed. S. Arber, and M. Evandrou. London: Jessica Kingsley.

Hubbard, P., A.F. Muhlenkamp, and N. Brown. 1984. The relationship between social support and self-care practices. *Nursing Res* 33:266–70.

Hunter, K.I., and M.W. Linn. 1979. Cultural and sex differences in dietary patterns of the urban elderly. *J Am Geri Soc* 27:359–63.

Iams, H.M., and S.H. Sandell. 1995. Changing social security benefits to reflect child-care years. *Fam Econ Nutr Rev* 8:49–52.

Kahn, R.L., and T.C. Antonucci. 1981. Convoys of social support: a life-course approach. In *Aging: Social change*, Ed. S.B. Kiesler, J.N. Morgan, and V.K. Oppenheimer. New York: Academic Press.

Kannel, W.B. 1995. Justification for management of blood lipids in the elderly. In *Nutritional assessment of elderly populations: Measure and function*, Ed. I.H. Rosenberg. New York: Raven Press.

Kant, A.K. 1996. Indexes of overall diet quality: A review. *J Am Diet Assoc* 96:785–91.

Karasik, R.J. 1989. Social interaction and integration among elderly, frail elderly and younger handicapped tenants of public senior housing. Master's thesis, University of Connecticut.

Katz, S., A.B. Ford, R.W. Moskowitz, B.A. Jackson, and M.W. Jaffe. 1963. The index of ADL: A standardized measure of biological and psychosocial function. *JAMA* 185:914–19.

Kavesh, W.N. 1986. Home care: Process, outcome, cost. In *Annual review of gerontology and geriatrics*. Vol. 6. Ed. C. Eisdorfer. New York: Springer.

Kaye, L.W., and A. Monk. 1991. Social relations in enriched housing for the aged: A case study. *J Hsg Elderly* 9:111–26.

Kelman, H.R., C. Thomas, and J.S. Tanaka. 1994. Longitudinal patterns of formal and informal social support in an urban elderly population. *Soc Sci Med* 38:905–14.

Kinard, J.D., and V.R. Kivett. 1983. Mealtime companionship and morale in the rural elderly. *J Nutr Eld* 3:3–15.

Kinsella, K. 1995. Aging and the family: Present and future demographic issues. In *Handbook of aging and the family*, Ed. R. Blieszner, and V.H. Bedford. Westport, CT: Greenwood Press.

Koehler, K.M., S.L. Pareo-Tubbeh, L.J. Romero, R.N. Baumgartner, and P.J. Garry. 1997. Folate nutrition and older adults: Challenges and opportunities. *J Am Diet Assoc* 97:167–73.

Kolasa, K.M., J.P. Mitchell, and A.C. Jobe. 1995. Food behaviors of southern rural community-living elderly. *Arch Fam Med* 4:844–48.

Kovar, M.G., G. Hendershot, and E. Mathis. 1989. Older people in the United States who receive help with basic activities of daily living. *Am J Pub Health* 79:778–79.

Kovar, M.G., J.D. Weeks, and W.F. Forbes. 1995. Prevalence of disability among older people: United States and Canada. *Vital and Health Statistics* 5(8).

Krause, N. 1989. Issues of measurement and analysis in studies of social support, aging and health. In *Aging, stress and health*, Ed. K.S. Markides, and C.L. Cooper. New York: John Wiley & Sons.

Krause, N., and E. Borawski-Clark. 1995. Social class differences in social support among older adults. *Gerontol* 35:498–508.

Krause, N., and K. Markides. 1990. Measuring social support among older adults. *Intl J Aging Hum Dev* 30:37–53.

Krause, N., and L.A. Wray. Psychosocial correlates of health and illness among minority elders. 1991. *Generations* 15(4):25–30.

Krebs-Smith, S.M., H. Smicklas-Wright, H.A. Guthrie, and J. Krebs-Smith. 1987. The effects of variety in food choices on dietary quality. *J Am Diet Assoc* 87:897–903.

Kriegsman, D.M.W., B.W.J.H. Penninx, and J.T.M. van Eijk. 1995. A criterion-based literature survey of the relationship between family support and incidence and course of chronic disease in the elderly. *Fam Syst Med* 13:39–68.

Krondl, M., D. Lau, M.A. Yurkiw, and P.H. Coleman. 1982. Food use and perceived food meanings of the elderly. *J Am Diet Assoc* 80:523–29.

Krueger, R.A. 1994. *Focus groups: A practical guide for applied research*. 2nd ed. Thousand Oaks, CA: Sage.

Kubena, K.S., W.A. McIntosh, M.B. Georghiades, and W.A. Landmann. 1991. Anthropometry and health in the elderly. *J Am Diet Assoc* 91:1402–07.

Kuczmarski, M.F. 1998. Nutritional status of older adults. In *Nutrition in aging*. 3rd ed. Ed. E.D. Schlenker. Boston: McGraw-Hill.

Kuller, L.H. 1997. Dietary fat and chronic disease: Epidemiologic overview. *J Am Diet Assoc* 97:S9–15.

Kwiterovich, P.O. 1997. The effect of dietary fat, antioxidants and pro-oxidants on blood lipids, lipoproteins and atherosclerosis. *J Am Diet Assoc* 97:S31–41.

La Rue, A., K.M. Koehler, S.J. Wayne, S.J. Chiulli, K.Y. Haaland, and P.J. Garry. 1997. Nutritional status and cognitive functioning in a normally aging sample: A 6-y reassessment. *Am J Clin Nutr* 65:20–29.

Landerman, R., L.K. George, R.T. Campbell, and D.G. Blazer. 1989. Alternative models of the stress buffering hypothesis. *Am J Comm Psychol* 17:625–42.

Lawton, M.P., and E.M. Brody. 1969. Assessment of older people: Self-maintaining and instrumental activities of daily living. *Gerontol* 9:179–86.

Learner, R.M., and V.R. Kivett. 1981. Discriminators of perceived dietary adequacy among the rural elderly. *J Am Diet Assoc* 78:330–37.

LeClerc, H.L., and M.E. Thornbury. 1983. Dietary intakes of Title III meal program recipients and nonrecipients. *J Am Diet Assoc* 83:573–77.

Lee, C.J., A.P. Warren, S. Godwin, J.C. Tsui, G. Perry, S.K. Hunt, R. Idris, R.S. Walker, H.F. Evans, F.E. Stigger, and S.S. Leftwich. 1993. Impact of special diets on the nutrient intakes of southern rural elderly. *J Am Diet Assoc* 93:186–88.

Linn, M.W. 1986. Elderly women's health and psychological adjustment: Life stressors and social support. In *Stress, social support and women*, Ed. S.E. Hobfoll. Washington, DC: Hemisphere.

Lipschitz, D.A., and J.V. White. 1991. *The development of an approach to nutrition screening for older Americans*. Washington, DC: Nutrition Screening Initiative.

Liu, K. 1994. Statistical issues related to semiquantitative food-frequency questionnaires. *Am J Clin Nutr* 59:262S-65.

Mares-Perlman, J.A., B.E.K. Klein, R. Klein, L.L. Ritter, M.R. Fisher, and J.L. Freudenheim. 1993. A diet history questionnaire ranks nutrient intakes in middle-aged and older men and women similarly to multiple food records. *J Nutr* 123:489–501.

McBride, J. 1995. Subtle larceny: Too little protein in elders. *Agr Res* 43:12–14.

McClelland, G.H., and C.M. Judd. 1993. Statistical difficulties of detecting interactions and moderator effects. *Psych Bull* 114:376–90.

McIntosh, W.A., and P.A. Shifflett. 1984. Influence of social support systems on dietary intake of the elderly. *J Nutr Eld* 4:5–18.

McIntosh, W.A, P.A. Shifflett, and J.S. Picou. 1989. Social support, stressful events, strain, dietary intake and the elderly. *Medical Care* 27:140–53.

Meunier, P.J., M.C. Chapuy, M.E. Arlot, and F. Duboeuf. 1995. Vitamin D and calcium: Their roles in pathophysiology and prevention of hip fractures. In *Nutritional assessment of elderly populations: Measure and function*, Ed. I.H. Rosenberg. New York: Raven Press.

Minten, V.K.A.M., M.R.H. Lowik, P. Deurenberg, and F.J. Kok. 1991 Inconsistent associations among anthropometric measurements in elderly Dutch men and women. *J Am Diet Assoc* 91:1408–12.

Mor-Barak, M.E., L.S. Miller, and L.S. Syme. 1991. Social networks, life events and health of the poor, frail elderly: A longitudinal study of the buffering versus the direct effect. *Fam Comm Health* 14:1–13.

Morgan, D.L. 1988. *Focus groups as qualitative research*. Newbury Park, CA: Sage.

Mowe, M., T. Bohmer, and E. Kindt. 1994. Reduced nutritional status in an elderly population (>70 y) is probable before disease and possibly contributes to the development of disease. *Am J Clin Nutr* 59:317–24.

Mullins, L.C., and M. Mushel. 1992. The existence and emotional closeness of relationships with children, friends and spouses: The effect on loneliness among older persons. *Res Aging* 14:448–70.

Murphy, S.P., A.F. Subar, and G. Block. 1990. Vitamin E intakes and sources in the United States. *Am J Clin Nutr* 52:361–67.

Nagi, S.Z. 1976. An epidemiology of disability among adults in the United States. *Milbank Mem Fund Q* 54:439–68.

Neyman, M.R., S. Zidenberg-Cherr, and R.B. McDonald. 1996. Effect of participation in congregate-site meal programs on nutritional status of the healthy elderly. *J Am Diet Assoc* 96:475–83.

Nieman, D.C., B.C. Underwood, K.M. Sherman, K. Arabatzis, J.C. Barbosa, M. Johnson, and T.D. Shultz. 1989. Dietary status of Seventh-Day Adventist vegetarian and non-vegetarian elderly women. *J Am Diet Assoc* 89:1763–69.

Noelker, L.S., and D.M. Bass. 1989. Home care for elderly persons: Linkages between formal and informal caregivers. *J Gerontol* 44:S63–70.

O'Hanlon, P., M.B. Kohrs, E. Hilderbrand, and J. Nordstrom. 1983. Socioeconomic factors and dietary intake of elderly Missourians. *J Am Diet Assoc* 82:646–53.

Packard, P.T., and R.P. Heaney. 1997. Medical nutrition therapy for patients with osteoporosis. *J Am Diet Assoc* 97:414–17.

Palmer, R.M. 1990. 'Failure to thrive' in the elderly: Diagnosis and management. *Geriatrics* 45:47–55.

Patterson, R.E., P.S. Haines, and B.M. Popkin. 1994. Diet quality index: Capturing a multidimensional behavior. *J Am Diet Assoc* 94:57–64.

Patterson, R.E., A.R. Kristal, R.J. Coates, F.A. Tylavsky, C. Ritenbaugh, L. Van Horn, A. Caggiula, and L. Snetselaar. 1996. Low-fat diet practices of older women: Prevalence and implications for dietary assessment. *J Am Diet Assoc* 96:670–79.

Payette, H., K. Gray-Donald, R. Cyr, and V. Boutier. 1995. Predictors of dietary intake in a functionally dependent elderly population in the community. *Am J Pub Health* 85:677–83.

Payne, R.L., and J.G. Jones. 1987. Measurement and methodological issues in social support. In *Stress and health: Issues in research methodology*, Ed. S.V. Kasl, and C.L. Cooper. New York: John Wiley.

Pearlin, L.I. 1989. The sociological study of stress. *J Health Soc Beh* 30:241–56.
Pearlin, L.I., M.A. Lieberman, E.G. Menaghan, and J.T. Mullan. 1981. The stress process. *J Health Soc Beh* 22:337–56.
Pedhazur, E.J. 1997. *Multiple regression in behavioral research: Explanation and prediction*. 3rd ed. New York: Harcourt Brace.
Pfeiffer, E. 1975. A short portable mental status questionnaire for the assessment of organic brain deficit in elderly patients. *J Am Geri Soc* 23:433–39.
Popkin, B.M., A.M. Siega-Riz, and P.S. Haines. 1996. A comparison of dietary trends among racial and socioeconomic groups in the United States. *N Engl J Med* 335:716–20.
Position of the American Dietetic Association. 1996. Nutrition, aging and the continuum of care. *J Am Diet Assoc* 96:1048–52.
Posner, B.E., C.G. Smigelski, and M.M. Krachenfels. 1987. Dietary characteristics and nutrient intake in an urban homebound population. *J Am Diet Assoc* 87:452–56.
Poulin, J.E. 1984. Age segregation and the interpersonal involvement and morale of the aged. *Gerontol* 24:266–69.
Ravussin, E., and P.A. Tataranni. 1997. Dietary fat and human obesity. *J Am Diet Assoc* 97:S42–46.
Reid, D.L., and J.E. Miles. 1977. Food habits and nutrient intakes of non-institutionalized senior citizens. *Can J Pub Health* 68:154–58.
Reuben, D.B., L.V. Rubenstein, S.H. Hirsch, and R.D. Hays. 1992. Value of functional status as a predictor of mortality: Results of a prospective study. *Am J Med* 93:663–69.
Revicki, D., and J. Mitchell. 1986. Social support factor structure in the elderly. *Res Aging* 8:232–48.
Rook, K.S. 1985. The functions of social bonds: Perspectives from research on social support, loneliness and social isolation. In *Social support: Theory, research and applications,* Ed. I.G. Sarason, and B.R. Sarason. Boston: Martinus Nijhoff.
Rook, K.S., and T.L. Schuster. 1996. Compensatory processes in the social networks of older adults. In *Handbook of social support and the family*, Ed. G.R. Pierce, B.R. Sarason, and I.G. Sarason. New York: Plenum Press.
Rosenberg, I.H., and J.W. Miller. 1992. Nutritional factors in physical and cognitive functions of elderly people. *Am J Clin Nutr* 55:1237S-43.

Rosenbloom, C.A., and F.J. Whittington. 1993. The effects of bereavement on eating behaviors and nutrient intakes in elderly widowed persons. *J Geront* 48:S223–29.

Roubenoff, R., G.E. Dallal, and P.W.F. Wilson. 1995. Predicting body fatness: The body mass index vs estimation by bioelectrical impedance. *Am J Pub Health* 85:726–28.

Rubinstein, R.L., J.E. Lubben, and J.E. Mintzer. 1994. Social isolation and social support: An applied perspective. *J Appl Gerontol* 13:58–72.

Russell, R.M. 1997. New views on the RDAs for older adults. *J Am Diet Assoc* 97:515–18.

Russell, R.M., and P.M. Suter. 1993. Vitamin requirements of elderly people: An update. *Am J Clin Nutr* 58:4–14.

Ryan, V.C., and M.E. Bower. 1989. Relationship of socioeconomic status and living arrangements to nutritional intake of the older person. *J Am Diet Assoc* 89:1805–07.

Sahyoun, N.R., P.F. Jacques, G.E. Dallal, and R.M. Russell. 1997. Nutrition Screening Initiative checklist may be a better awareness/educational tool than a screening one. *J Am Diet Assoc* 97:760–64.

Saluter, A.F. 1996. *Current population reports: Marital status and living arrangements, March 1994.* Series P20–484, Washington DC: U.S. Government Printing Office.

Salvini, S., D.J. Hunter, L. Sampson, M.J. Stampfer, G.A. Colditz, B. Rosner, and W.C. Willett. 1989. Food-based validation of a dietary questionnaire: The effects of week-to-week variation in food consumption. *Inter J Epidem* 18:858–67.

SAS Institute Inc. 1996. Statistical Analysis System (SAS) Software Version 6.09. Cary NC.

Sauer, W.J., and R.T. Coward. 1985. The role of social support networks in the care of the elderly. In *Social support networks and the care of the elderly: Theory, research and practice,* Ed. W.J. Sauer, and R.T. Coward. New York: Springer.

Schafer, R.B., and P.M. Keith. 1982. Social-psychological factors in the dietary quality of married and single elderly. *J Am Diet Assoc* 81:30–34.

Schafer, R.B., P.M. Keith, and E. Schafer. 1994. The effects of marital interaction, depression and self-esteem on dietary self-efficacy among married couples. *J Applied Soc Psych* 24:2209–22.

Schlenker, E.D. 1998. *Nutrition in aging.* 3$^{rd}$ ed. New York: McGraw-Hill.

Schlicker, S.A., S.A. Atkinson, I.H. Rosenberg, and J.T. Dwyer. 1997. Dietary reference intakes for calcium and related nutrients. Presentation at the 80th Annual Meeting of the American Dietetic Association, Boston, MA.

Seelbach, W.C. 1978. Correlates of aged parents' filial responsibility expectations and realizations. *Fam Coord* 27:341–50.

Seeman, T.E., and L.F. Berkman. 1988. Structural characteristics of social networks and their relationship with social support in the elderly: Who provides support. *Soc Sci Med* 26:737–49.

Seidel, J., S. Friese, and D.C. Leonard. 1995. The Ethnograph v4.0: A program for the analysis of text based data. Qualis Research Associates, Salt Lake City, UT.

Sem, S.W., M. Nes, K. Engedal, J.I. Pedersen, and K. Trygg. 1988. An attempt to identify and describe a group of non-institutionalized elderly with the lowest nutrient score. *Compr Gerontol A* 2:60–66.

Sheehan, N.W. 1986. Informal support among the elderly in public senior housing. *Gerontol* 26:171–75.

Shepherd, S.K., and C.L. Achterberg. 1992. Qualitative research methodology: Data collection, analysis, interpretation and verification. In *Research: Successful approaches,* Ed. E.R. Monson. Mexico: American Dietetic Association.

Shifflett, P.A., and W.A. McIntosh. 1986. Food habits and future time: An exploratory study of age-appropriate food habits among the elderly. *Intl J Aging Hum Dev* 24:2–17.

Siegel, J.S. 1993. *A generation of change: A profile of America's older population.* New York: Russel Sage.

Slesinger, D.P., M. McDivitt, and F.M. O'Donnell. 1980. Food patterns in an urban population: Age and sociodemographic correlates. *J Gerontol* 35:432–41.

Smiciklas-Wright, H., D.J. Lago, V. Bernardo, and J.L. Beard. 1990. Nutritional assessment of homebound rural elderly. *J Nutr* 120:1535–37.

Smith, L.A., L.G. Branch, P.A. Scherr, T. Wetle, D.A. Evans, L. Hebert, and J.O. Taylor. 1990. Short-term variability of measures of physical function in older people. *J Am Geri Soc* 38:993–98.

Smucker, R., G. Block, L. Coyle, A. Harvin, and L. Kessler. 1989. A dietary and risk factor questionnaire and analysis system for personal computers. *Am J Epidem* 129:445–49.

Spradley, J.P. 1979. *The ethnographic interview.* New York: Holt, Rinehart & Winston.

Stein, S., M.W. Linn, E. Slater, and E.M. Stein. 1989. Future concerns and recent life events of elderly community residents. In *Stressful life events*, Ed. T.W. Miller. Madison, CT: International University Press.

Stoller, E.P., and K.L. Pugliesi. 1989. The transition to the caregiving role: A panel study of helpers of elderly people. *Res Aging* 11:312–30.

Struyk, R.J., D.B. Page, S. Newman, M. Carroll, M. Ueno, B. Cohen, and P. Wright. 1989. *Providing supportive services to the frail elderly in federally assisted housing*. Washington, DC: Urban Institute Press.

Suitor, J.J., and K. Pillemer. 1993. Support and interpersonal stress in the social networks of married daughters caring for parents with dementia. *J Gerontol* 48:S1–8.

Tabachnick, B.G., and L.S. Fidell. 1989. *Using multivariate statistics*. 2$^{nd}$ ed. New York: Harper and Row.

Taylor-Davis, S.A., and H. Smiciklas-Wright. 1993. The quality of survey data obtained from elderly adults. *J Nutr Eld* 13:11–21.

Tesch, R. 1990. *Qualitative research: Analysis types and software tools*. New York: Falmer Press.

Thoits, P.A. 1982. Conceptual, methodological and theoretical problems in studying social support as a buffer against life stress. *J Health Soc Beh* 23:145–59.

Toner, H.M. 1987. An exploratory investigation of self-actualization, social support and dietary quality in later adulthood. Ph.D. diss., Florida Atlantic University.

Toner, H.M., and J.D. Morris. 1992. A social-psychological perspective of dietary quality in later adulthood. *J Nutr Eld* 11:35–53.

Travis, S.S. 1995. Families and formal networks. In *Handbook of aging and the family*, Ed. R. Blieszner and V.H. Bedford. Westport, CT: Greenwood Press.

Troll, L.E. 1994. Family-embedded vs. family-deprived oldest-old: A study of contrasts. *Intl J Aging Hum Dev* 38:51–63.

U.S. Bureau of the Census. 1992. *1990 Census of population: General population characteristics, CT*. Washington, DC: U.S. Government Printing Office.

U.S. Bureau of the Census. 1993. *1990 Census of population: Social and economic characteristics, CT*. Washington, DC: U.S. Government Printing Office.

U.S. Bureau of the Census. 1996. *Current population reports, special studies: 65+ in the United States*. P23–190, Washington, DC: U.S. Government Printing Office.

U.S. Department of Agriculture (USDA), Agricultural Research Service, Dietary Guidelines Advisory Committee. 1995. *Report of the dietary guidelines committee on the dietary guidelines for Americans*. Washington, DC: USDA.

U.S. Department of Health and Human Services. 1988. *The surgeon general's report on nutrition and health: summary and recommendations*. DHHS No. 88–50211 Washington, DC: U.S. Government Printing Office.

U.S. Department of Health and Human Services, Office of the Secretary. 1996. Annual update of the HHS poverty guidelines. Federal Register 61(43):8286–87.

Vailas, L., L. Russo, C. Rankin, and S. Nitzke. 1997. Nutrition risk in Wisconsin elderly meal program participants. *Gerontol Nutr Newsletter* Spr:5–6.

Van Zandt, S. 1986. Nutritional impact of congregate meals programs. *J Nutr Eld* 5:31–43.

Vaughn, S., J.S. Schumm, and J. Sinagub. 1996. *Focus group interviews in education and psychology*. Thousand Oaks, CA: Sage.

Vaux, A. 1988. *Social support: Theory, research and intervention*. New York: Praeger.

Walker, D., and R.E. Beauchene. 1991. The relationship of loneliness, social isolation and physical health to dietary adequacy of independently living elderly. *J Am Diet Assoc* 91:300–04.

Weisburger, J.H. 1997. Dietary fat and risk of chronic disease: Mechanistic insights from experimental studies. *J Am Diet Assoc* 97:S16–23.

Weiss, R.S. 1994. *Learning from strangers: The art and method of qualitative interview studies*. New York: Free Press.

Wellman, B., and S. Wortley. 1989. Brothers' keepers: Situating kinship relations in broader networks of social support. *Soc Perspec* 32:273–306.

Westenbrink, S., M.R.H. Lowik, K.F.A.M. Hulshof, and C. Kistemaker. 1989. Effect of household size on nutritional patterns among the Dutch elderly. *J Am Diet Assoc* 89:793–99.

Wheaton, B. 1985. Models for the stress-buffering functions of coping resources. *J Health Soc Beh* 26:352–64.

White, J.V. 1991. *Risk factors associated with poor nutritional status in older Americans*. Washington, DC: Nutrition Screening Initiative.

Witte, D.J., J.D. Skinner, and B.R. Carruth. 1991. Relationship of self-concept to nutrient intake and eating patterns in young women. *J Am Diet Assoc* 91:1068–73.
Wolf, D.A. 1994. The elderly and their kin: Patterns of availability and access. In *Demography of aging,* Ed. L.G. Martin, and S.H. Preston. Washington, DC: National Academy Press.
Zipp, A., and C.A. Holcomb. 1992. Living arrangements and nutrient intakes of healthy women age 65 and older: A study in Manhattan, Kansas. *J Nutr Eld* 11:1–18.
Zulkifli, S.N., and S.M. Yu. 1992. The food frequency method for dietary assessment. *J Am Diet Assoc* 92:681–85.

# Author Index

Abel, E., 74, 83, 99, 168
Abernathy, R., 56
Achterberg, C., 30
Ahmed, F., 125, 126, 128
Aiken, L., 144, 148, 150, 155, 161
Akiyama, H., 3, 28, 112, 115, 181
Allender, P., 130
Antonucci, T., 3, 4, 7, 23, 26, 28, 112, 114, 115, 169, 181
Armstrong, M., 115, 181

Badger, M., 12
Barrera, M., 15, 23, 26, 140, 170
Bass, D., 115
Beauchene, R., 9, 11, 20, 113, 121, 135, 145, 170
Berkman, L., 10, 12
Betts, N., 20
Bianchetti, A., 7, 20, 145–46, 170
Bidlack, W., 123, 125, 126, 128
Biegel, D., 113
Bisogni, C., 4, 11, 73
Blalock, H., 9
Block, G., 41, 43, 46, 117, 120, 121–22, 126, *127*, 136
Bloom, J., 3

Bohmer, T., 58
Borawski-Clark, E., 28
Bower, M., 7, 28
Bowling, A., 3
Broadhead, W., 3
Brody, E., 36, 44, 52, *142*
Brown, N., 8

Calasanti, T., 7, 12
Campbell, W., 123–24
Carpenter, B., 3, 13, 51
Carruth, B., 9
Chappell, N., 12, 115
Chiriboga, D., 18–20
Clancy, K., 12
Coe, R., 3, 6, 11, 12
Cohen, N., 11, 12
Cohen, S., 21, 27, 88, 147
Coulston, A., 121
Coward, R., 6
Craig, L., 121
Crimmins, E., 52, 53, 146
Crohan, S., 114, 169
Cummings, S., 41, 136
Cutler, J., 130
Cutrona, C., 12

Dakof, G., 74, 88, 114, 168
Davies, L., 3
Davis, M., 8, 10
Dawson-Hughes, B., 128
de Castro, J., 11
Dean, A., 45
Duffy, V., 46
Dunlap, W., 148
Dwyer, J., 51, 146

Eggebeen, D., 114
Ely, D., 131
Ernst, N., 130
Evans, W., 123

Falk, L., 4, 11, 73
Fanelli, M., 120
Farkas, K., 113
Farquhar, M., 3
Fey-Yensan, N., 41
Fidell, L., 145, 166
Fillenbaum, G., 34, 35
Finney, J., 148
Fischer, J., 58
Fitti, J., 53
Fogler-Levitt, E., 113
Follmann, D., 130
Forbes, W., 54–55
Friese, S., 31, 37
Frongillo, E., 8, 20
Fulton, J., 54–55

Galanos, A., 21, 56
George, L., 18–19, 23
Gibson, R., 133
Golant, S., 51, 63
Goldsteen, K., 115, 181

Gottlieb, B., 33, 35, 37, 74, 82, 168
Gray-Donald, K., 3
Greenbaum, T., 29, 31
Grundy, E., 3
Guigoz, Y., 128
Guse, L., 115
Guthrie, H., 44, 135, *143*

Haboubi, N., 42, 55
Haines, P., 41, 44, 121, 133, 135, 136, *143*
Ham, R., 58
Hanson, B., 9, 11, 12, 14, 42, 60, *61*, 174
Hansson, R., 3, 13, 51
Harris, T., 21, 53
Harrison, G., 130
Hartman, A., 41
Heaney, R., 128
Heller, K., 9, 11, 12, 14–15
Hellman, E., 115
Hendershot, G., 52
Hendricks, J., 7, 12
Hinrichsen, G., 51
Hogan, D., 114
Holcomb, C., 7, 11, 58, 121, 126
Horwath, C., 8, 11
Howarth, G., 68
Hubbard, P., 8
Hudson, P., 42, 55
Hunter, K., 10, 20, 28, 145, 170

Iams, H., 51

Jobe, A., 7, 20
Johnson, M., 58
Jones, J., 177

*Author Index*

Judd, C., 148, 155, 157, 161, 163

Kahn, R., 26
Kannel, W., 137
Kant, A., 133, 134, 156
Karasik, R., 51
Katz, S., 36, 44, 52, *142*
Kavesh, W., 115
Kaye, L., 51
Keith, P., 6, 9, 10
Kelman, H., 115
Kemery, E., 148
Kinard, J., 11
Kindt, E., 58
Kinsella, K., 28, 62
Kivett, V., 9, 11, 12
Knutson, K., 3
Koehler, K., 129
Kolasa, K., 7, 20
Kovar, M., 52, 53, 54–55
Krachenfels, M., 7
Krause, N., 3, 15, 26, 28, 164
Krebs–Smith, S., 135
Kriegsman, D., 12, 14
Krondl, M., 73
Krueger, R., 29–30
Kubena, K., *58*
Kuczmarski, M., 56, 137
Kuller, L., 130
Kwiterovich, P., 131

La Rue, A., 125
Landerman, R., 163, 170
Lawton, M., 36, 44, 52, *142*
Learner, R., 9, 11, 12
LeClerc, H., 7, 11, *98*
Lee, C., *98*
Leonard, D., 31, 37

Linn, M., 10, 19–20, 28, 145, 170
Lipschitz, D., 42, 59, 181
Liu, K., 136
Lubben, J., 7, 12

Mansbach, W., 9, 11, 12, 14–15
Mares-Perlman, J., 41, 121, 125, *127*, 136
Markides, K., 27
Mathis, E., 52
Mattisson, I., 9, 11, 12, 14, 60, 174
McBride, J., 123–24
McClelland, G., 148, 155, 157, 161, 163
McDivitt, M., 7
McDonald, R., 4, 113, 125
McIntosh, W., 10, 12, 16–17
Meunier, P., 137
Miles, J., 7
Miller, D., 3, 6, 11
Miller, J., 3
Miller, L., 180
Minten, V., *58*
Mintzer, J., 7, 12
Mitchell, J., 7, 12, 20
Monk, A., 51
Mor-Barak, M., 180
Morgan, D., 29–30
Morris, J., 15–16
Mowe, M., 58
Muhlenkamp, A., 8
Mullins, L., 10
Murphy, S., 126
Mushel, M., 10

Nagi, S., 36, 44, 52, *142*
Neyman, M., 4, 113, 125, *127*
Nieman, D., 125, *127*

Noelker, L., 115

O'Donnell, F., 7
O'Hanlon, P., 28
Ostergren, P., 42, 60, *61*

Packard, P., 128
Palmer, R., 3
Pathy, M., 42, 56
Patterson, R., 41, 44, 121, 133, 136, *143*
Payette, H., 7, 11, 19, *58*, 112
Payne, R., 177
Pearlin, L., 12, 18–19, 27
Pedhazur, E., 16, 27, 144, 145, 148, 150, 176
Penninx, B., 12, 14
Pfeiffer, E., 34
Picou, J., 10, 16–17
Pillemer, K., 113
Popkin, B., 41, 44, 121, 133, 135, 136, *143*
Posner, B., 7, *127*
Poulin, J., 51
Pugliesi, K., 112

Ralston, P., 11, 12
Ramsay, T., 15, 26
Ravussin, E., 130
Reid, D., 7
Reuben, D., 52
Revicki, D., 12
Rook, K., 4–6, 8, 10, 13, 16, 18, 24, 114, 115, *141*, 169, 173, 174, 177
Rosenberg, I., 3
Rosenbloom, C., 19, 28
Roubenoff, R., 58

Rubinstein, R., 7, 12
Russell, R., 125–26, 128–29
Ryan, V., 7, 28

Sahyoun, N., 59
Saito, Y., 52, 53, 146
Saluter, A., 48
Salvini, S., 136, 176
Sandell, S., 51
Sandler, I., 15, 26
Sauer, W., 6
Schafer, E., 6
Schafer, R., 6, 9, 10
Scheer, J., 44, 135, *143*
Schlenker, E., 123, 125, 126, 128, 131
Schlicker, S., 128
Schumm, J., 29
Schuster, T., 114–15, 169
Seelbach, W., 28
Seeman, T., 10, 12
Seidel, J., 31, 37
Sem, S., 7, 10, 11, *58*
Sheehan, N., 51
Shepherd, S., 30
Shifflett, P., 10, 12, 16–17, *98*
Siega-Riz, A., 135
Siegel, J., 47, 51, 135
Sinagub, J., 29
Skinner, J., 9
Slesinger, D., 7
Smiciklas-Wright, H., 7, 28, 175–78
Smigelski, C., 7
Smith, L., 52
Smucker, R., 44, 45, 136
Sobal, J., 4, 11, 73
Spradley, J., 34

Steen, B., 9, 11, 12, 14, 60, 174
Stein, S., 67
Stevenhagen, K., 120
Stewart, C., 115
Stoller, E., 112
Struyk, R., 175
Subar, A., 121–22, 126
Suitor, J., 113
Suter, P., 126
Syme, L., 180

Tabachnick, B., 145, 166
Tanaka, J., 115
Tataranni, P., 130
Taylor, S., 74, 88, 114, 168
Taylor-Davis, S., 175–78
Tesch, R., 38
Thoits, P., 23, 177
Thomas, C., 115
Thornbury, M., 7, 11
Toner, H., 15–16, 17, 99, 135
Travis, S., 114
Troll, L., 114
Turner, H., 7

Vailas, L., 59
van Eijk, J., 12, 14
Van Zandt, S., 4
Vaughn, S., 29
Vaux, A., 23
Vivian, V., 20
Voss, A., 121

Wadsworth, N., 113
Walker, D., 9, 11, 20, 113, 121, *127*, 135, 145, 170
Wang, W., 123, 125, 126, 128
Weeks, J., 54–55

Weisburger, J., 131
Weiss, R., 25, 32, 34
Wellman, B., 23, 114
West, S., 144, 148, 150, 155, 161
Westenbrink, S., 8, *98*
Wheaton, B., 140, 147, 177
White, J., 3, 7, 42, 56, 58, 59, 181
Whittington, F., 19, 28
Wills, T., 21, 27, 88, 147
Witte, D., 9
Wolf, D., 28
Wortley, S., 23, 114
Wray, L., 3

Yu, S., 136

Zidenberg-Cherr, S., 4, 113, 125
Zipp, A., 7, 11, 58, 126, *127*
Zulkifli, S., 136

# Subject Index

accompaniment, 76, 77–78, 82, 101, 106–7
acknowledgement, 94
Activities of Daily Living. *See* functional status
advice, 76, 78, 83, 91, 94, 174
alcohol, 130–31
anthropometrics, 42–43, 56–58
antioxidant, 126, 131
appetite, 11, 17, 19
arthritis. *See* illness, chronic
ascorbic acid, 122, 131, 133
availability, 78, 168–71

barriers to good nutrition, 66–74, 82
Body Mass Index:
    and functional status, 21
    and health, 58
    and receipt of support, 88, 116
    reference criteria, 56
    and satisfaction with support, 95, 97, 110, 170
    and social anchorage, 12, 174
    of subjects, 56–58

bone loss, 127–28. *See also* osteoporosis
breakfast, 117
buffering model, 139–40, 144
    Diet Quality Index as outcome, 148–52, 160, 163
    Mean Adequacy Ratio as outcome, 153–60, 160, 163
    statistical equations, 144, 147
    summary of findings, 164–66, 171

calcium, 122, 126–29, 133, *134*
calories:
    intake of, 121, *122*, 123, 156
    and magnesium, 128
    and Mean Adequacy Ratio, 156
    top food contributors of, 120–21
    and zinc, 125
cancer. *See* illness, chronic
card sort, 32, 34, 35
cardiovascular disease. *See* illness, chronic

census data, 47–48, 50, 51, 54–55, 62
children, 11, 19, 68. *See also* daughters; sons
cholesterol, 130–31, *134*
cliques, 108–9
companionship:
   in contrast to emotional support, 13, 23
   functions of, 4–6, 114
   influence on diet, 8–10, 174
   mealtime, 11, 60, 68, 108, 113
conditional effects, 144, 159, 172–75
constipation, 70
contacts, 11, 51
control, 4–6. *See also* integration, social
controlling. *See* social support, nutrition related: misguided
cooking, 32, 68–69, 108
coping, 21, 51–52
core foods, 120
crisis help, 114
cross-sectional design, 115, 175

daughters:
   and diet support, 78–80, 91, 94, 99
   and food procurement support, 76–78, 104–7
   in-law, 95
   and misguided support, 81
   nutrition education for, 178
demographics, 47–51
dentition, 70–71
diabetes. *See* illness, chronic
diet, modified:
   appropriateness of, 88, 98
   as barrier to good nutrition, 70–71
   comparison, physician- and self-prescribed, 87
   and emotional support, 79–80, 91, 99
   and informational support, 78–79, 91, 99
   occurrence and types of, 86–88, 98
   operational definition for, 44
   reasons for, 70, 73, 86
   *See also* weight
diet, physician-prescribed:
   and likelihood of support, 88, 99, 169
   occurrence and types of, 87–88
diet quality, 132–33, 136–38
   in buffering model, 143–44, 148–52, 153–60
   Diet Quality Index, 133–36, 150
   food pattern, 121
   and functional status, 20–21, 145–46, 170
   Mean Adequacy Ratio, 133–36, 159
   nutrient intakes, 121–29
   as outcome measure, 43–44
   and social isolation, 174
   *See also* Dietary Guidelines for Americans; Recommended Dietary Allowance
diet recommendations, 121, 137–38
diet records, 9, 136

## Subject Index

Dietary Guidelines for Americans, 122, 129–32
Dietary Reference Intakes, 128
dietitian, 79, 91
directive, 76, 78, 83, 91, 94, 174
disability. *See* functional status
disease. *See* illness, acute; illness, chronic
distraction, 80
doctor. *See* physician, as helper

eating out, 69, 166
education, nutrition:
    formal providers of, 79, 91, 99
    recommendations for, 178–81
education, years schooling:
    and diet quality, 135–36
    and receipt of support, 88, 116
    and satisfaction with support, 95, 97, 110
    of subjects, 48
emotional closeness, 9, 10–11
emotional support. *See* support, emotional
empathy, 80, 94
encouragement, 76, 79–80, 91, 94
energy. *See* calories; weight

Family Nutrition Program, 25
fat, dietary, 130–32, 133–34, 178
fiber, 88, 130–32
5 A Day campaign, 137
focus groups, 29–31, 66, 108–9
folate, 122, 128–29, 133
food:
    allergies and insensitivities, 70–71, 108
    cost, 67, 69, 73, 74, 108

    gifts of, 104
    groupings, 120
    issues, of subjects, 69–71
    labels, 68
    preferences, 69–70, 73, 108, 113
    procurement of, 66–69, 76–77, 100–9, 179–83
    security, 67, 72, 101
Food Behavior Inventory, 41
food frequency questionnaire, 41, 46, 136–37, 117–38, 176
food patterns:
    change in, as stressor, 20–21
    factors that influence, 4, 73, 86
    and functional status, 20
    nutrition education to improve, 178
    of subjects, 117–21, 136–37
friends:
    and appetite, 16–17
    and diet support, 80, 91, 94
    and food procurement support, 77, 78, 104–7, 112
    as potential stress, 19
functional status:
    in buffering model, 143–44
    and diet quality, 145–46, 170
    and food procurement support, 101–6, 112, 115, 161, 179–83
    and meal programs, 108–9, 113
    measurement of, 35, *36*, 52–53, *142*, 176
    and receipt of support, 88, 116, 150, 160
    as recruitment criteria, 28

and relation to health, 51–53, 124
and satisfaction with support, 95, 97, 110
as stressor on diet quality, 20–21, 72, 77, 168–71
of subjects, 52–55
*See also* buffering model

gender, 8, 10–11, 18, 28, 48, 50–51
generalizability, 47, 55, 60, 62–63, 74, 175
geographic area, 39, 48, *49*
grandchildren, 81, 107
graying of America, 62
grocery shopping. *See* food: procurement

health, self-rated:
  and diet quality, 135–36
  and likelihood diet support, 88
  and satisfaction with support, 95, 97, 110
  of subjects, 51, *52*.
  *See also* illness, chronic
helping behaviors:
  coding definition, 37
  described by key informants, 74–80
  described by other groups, 82–83
  related stressors, 82
  *See also* social support, nutrition-related
hierarchical-compensatory model, 114–15

hierarchy of support providers, 115, 169
home health aide, 77, 104–7
housing, government subsidized:
  rent in, 50, 63
  as selection criteria, 27–28, 38–39
  and social support, 51, 175
  variability in, 45–46, 63
hypertension. *See* illness, chronic

illness, acute:
  as concern, 72
  and immune function, 131–32
  and protein, 123
  and vitamin B6, 125
  and zinc, 125
illness, chronic:
  and calcium, 128
  Diet Quality Index, as risk indicator for, 133–34
  Dietary Guidelines, to reduce, 130–32
  and folate, 129
  and magnesium, 128
  and protein, 123–24
  as reason for diet change, 70
  in subjects, 62, 51–52
income, estimated from rent:
  and diet quality, 135
  and receipt of support, 88, 116
  and satisfaction with support, 95, 97, 110
  of subjects 50–51, 63
independence:
  emotional, 99
  instrumental, 101
  loss of, 47–48, 132

to maintain, 137–38, 179–181
and reciprocity, 164–66
informational support. *See*
support, informational
instrumental support. *See* support,
instrumental
integration, social:
contrasted with social support,
13, 173–76
functions of, 5–6
influence on diet, 10–12, 16

interaction, statistical. *See*
statistical effects
interviewers, 37, 38, 40, 110
interviews:
key informant, 34–35
pilot, 25–27
structured, 38, 40, 91, 176
Inventory of Socially Supportive
Behaviors, 15, 26
iron, 122, 133
isolation, social:
and diet quality, 3, 174
and social integration, 4, 6
*See also* social anchorage
issue statements, 31–*33*, 35, 73–74, *75*

joint relation, 144, 147, 148–49,
150, 157

kin. *See* social support, general:
formal/informal

lean body mass, 123–24
leftovers, 69
life satisfaction, and diet, 9

living arrangement:
influence on diet, 7–8
as proxy for social support, 7
of subjects, 49–51
*See also* housing, government
subsidized
living arrangement, duration of:
and diet quality, 136
and receipt of support, 88, 116
and satisfaction with support,
95, 110
loneliness, 9, 113
Longitudinal Study on Aging, 21,
54–55
long-term support, 114

magnesium, *122*, 128, 133
main effects. *See* statistical effects:
direct
marital status:
as proxy for social support,
10–11, 14
of subjects, 48
widowhood, 19–20, 28
meal:
as defined by subjects, 68, 69
invitation, as type of support,
104
meal programs:
DETERMINE scores of
participants, 59
and diet quality, 166
as source of support, 104, 108,
112–13
medications, 60, 120, 128
mental health:
effect on diet, 71
measurement of, 34–35, 39

and vitamin B6, 125
model of social relationships and diet:
    alternate models, 23, 176–79
    proposed, 4–6, 7, 21
    statistically tested, 171, 174
    *See also* buffering model
moderator model. *See* buffering model
motivation, 68, 99, 176
Multidimensional Functional Assessment Instrument, 20–21, 34–36
muscle. *See* lean body mass

National Cancer Institute. *See* food frequency questionnaire
National Food Consumption Survey, 8, 120, 135
National Health and Nutrition Examination Survey, 8, 10–11, 21, 46, 56, 120, 126, 128, 135
National Health Interview Survey, 121–22, 126
network:
    convoy approach, 26
    structural properties, 4, 10–12, 18
niacin, 122
nutrient density, 120, 156. *See also* diet quality
nutrient intakes, 121–29, 131. *See also individual nutrients, ie.* calories; iron, *etc.*
Nutrition Screening Initiative, 42, 58–60, 181
Nutrition Social Support Questionnaire, 42

nutritional risk:
    of chronic disease, 133–34
    stress and support as indicators of, 181–84
    *See also* Body Mass Index; Nutrition Screening Initiative

obesity. *See* Body Mass Index; illness, chronic
obligation, 10, 115
operational definitions, *142–43*, 145
osteoporosis, 127–28, 131–32, 137, 178, 179
outcome measures, *43*, 43–45

perceptions:
    of nutrition problems, 27, 29, 66
    understanding, 82, 182
    *See also* barriers to good nutrition
physician, as helper, 78–80, 91, 94
pilot studies, 25–27, 34
polyunsaturated fatty acids, 126
population growth, 47, 62
poverty, 50, 62
    and Body Mass Index, 58
    and food cost, 67, 74
    and vitamin B6, 125–26
processed food, 67, *87*
protein:
    in Diet Quality Index, *134*
    intake of, 122–24
    in Mean Adequacy Ratio, 133
    and stress, 19, 123
    and vitamin B6, 125
    and zinc, 125

Subject Index        *241*

public programs:
  funding for, 62
  inflexibility of, 66, 108–9
  recommendations for, 3–4, 178–84
  *See also* meal programs

qualitative methods:
  depth interviews, 26, 32–38
  focus groups, 29–31
  follow-up interviews, 31–32

reciprocal help:
  and receipt of support, 88, 116
  and satisfaction with support, 95, 97, 110
reciprocity, 15, 164–66, 180
Recommended Dietary Allowance, 123, 137
  as basis for Mean Adequacy Ratio, 133
  subject intakes, compared to, 122–29
  suggested revisions to, 128–29
  *See also* Dietary Reference Intakes
recruitment, 29, 31, 34, 38–39
referral, 80, 91
regression, statistical:
  hierarchical, 147–48
  nonlinear, 161, 176
  ordinary least squares, 145, 147
research, nonexperimental, 27, 144, 155, 157, 176
riboflavin, *122*, 128–29, 133
role-model, 80, 94
roles, 6, 10, 114–15

routine, 69

salt. *See* sodium
satisfaction:
  in absence of support, 27, 95
  in buffering model, 163–65
  with diet support, 95–98, 170
  with food procurement support, 109–11, 170, 172, 173
  with social contact, 12
screening data. *See* statistical: diagnostics
self-disclosure, 76, 80, 83, 91, 94, 174
self-esteem, 4–6, 9–10
Senior Nutrition Awareness Project, 38–39, 91
Short Portable Mental Status Questionnaire, 34–35
snacking, 69, 71
social anchorage:
  measurement of, 42
  and receipt of support, 88, 116
  and satisfaction with support, 95, 97, 110
  of subjects, 60, *61*
  *See also* isolation, social
social support, for diet:
  misguided, 174
  providers of, 88–91
  receipt of, 88, 99
  satisfaction with, 95–98
  types of, 91–94
  *See also* support, emotional; support, informational
social support, for food procurement:

in buffering model, 143–44,
148–52, 153–60
case comparison, 100–1
programmatic, 107–9, 179–83
providers of, 104–7, 112, 150,
159
receipt of, 106, 111
satisfaction with, 109–11, 163–
65
types of, 101–4, 159–61
*See also* support, instrumental
social support, general, 3–6, 13–18
alternate frameworks, 23–24,
177
formal/informal, 4, 15, 62, 115
functions of, 4, 12, 13, 114
high helper, 173
social support, nutrition related:
absence of, 74, 82, 112
adequacy, 173
formal/informal, 100, 114, 169
measurement of, 42
misguided, 37, 81–82, 173
operational definition, 44–45
perceived, 26
*See also* helping behaviors
sodium, 122, 130–32, *134*
sons:
and diet support, 94
and food procurement support,
104–7
and misguided support, 81
special diet. *See* diet, modified
stages of change theory, 178
statistical:
analyses, summarized, 45
diagnostics, 145, 161, 166

error, 16, 136–37, 146, 166,
175–79
interpretation, 144, 148, 177–
178
model. *See* buffering model
power, 38, 155, 166
significance, 157, 163
variables, *142–43*, 143, 145,
148
statistical effects, 18
direct, 17, 144, 177
indirect, 9
interactive, 16–17, 143–44,
147, 157
stress, 18–21, 180–83
chronic, 20–21
daily hassles, 19, 69
financial, 17, 19, 67
life events, 19–20, 69
nutrition barriers, *33*
and protein, 19, 123
and salt sensitivity, 131
and social support, 6, 13, 16,
27, 65–66
subjects:
attrition of, 39, 45
description of, 48–63
limitations of, 175
in pilot, 25–26
selection criteria for, 27–28, 39
*See also* recruitment
summary scores, 139, 166
supplements, 117, 123, 136, 137
support, emotional:
frequency and providers of,
91–94, 113–15, 168–71
misguided, 173–76
in model, 13–15

## Subject Index

nutrition educators to provide, 178–81
in schema of helping behaviors, 76, 79–80, 168
support, informational:
frequency and providers of, 91–94, 114–15, 168–71
misguided, 173
in model, 13–14
nutrition educators to provide, 178–81
in schema of helping behaviors, 76, 78–79, 168
support, instrumental:
and availability, 78
and diet quality, 164–66
frequency and providers of, 113–15, 168–71
in model, 13–15
in schema of helping behaviors, 76–77, 168

task-specific model, 114–15, 169
taste:
changes, 70, 125
preferences. *See* food: preferences
technical help, 114
textual analysis, 26, 31, 37–38, 73–74
thiamin, *122*, 133
time, 45, 108
transportation, 66, 76, 101, *107*, 108, 179
24-hour diet recall, 9, 15, 135

vitamin A, *122*, 128–29, 131–32, 133

vitamin B6, *122*, 125, 128–29, 133
vitamin D, *122*, 127, 132
vitamin E, 122, 126, 131
vitamins/minerals, 117, 123. *See also* diet quality

weight:
dieting, to lose, 71, 79–80
status, of subjects, 56–58, 123
underweight, 58
*See also* Body Mass Index
widowhood, 19–20, 28

zinc, *122*, 125, 133

For Product Safety Concerns and Information please contact our EU
representative  GPSR@taylorandfrancis.com
Taylor & Francis Verlag GmbH, Kaufingerstraße 24, 80331 München, Germany

www.ingramcontent.com/pod-product-compliance
Lightning Source LLC
Chambersburg PA
CBHW070559300426
44113CB00010B/1323